Sunday Times Hu

'A funny, poignant snap

Radio Times

'The perfect surgical stocking filler. Jokes galore. This little book will no doubt cheer up the many readers who find it under their tree'   *The Times*

'Will have you crying with laughter'

Good Housekeeping

'Beyond hilarious . . . A small but perfectly formed follow-up to *This is Going to Hurt*, this Christmas-themed delight continues to capture the dark humour and dedicated work of NHS professionals everywhere'   *Stylist*

'Contains Kay's unique alchemy of medical insight and cynical wit'   *Daily Mirror*

'Hilarious and heartbreaking'   *Irish Times*

'Kay's fans will be delighted to discover that it is entirely as revolting, funny and moving as the first' inews.co.uk

'Matchless stories . . . funny, disgusting and moving'

Guardian

Adam Kay is an award-winning comedian and author of the multi-million-copy bestseller *This is Going to Hurt*. He previously worked as a junior doctor, which is hopefully clear by now. He lives in Oxfordshire.

ADAM KAY

Twas the Nightshift
Before Christmas

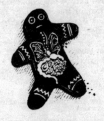

PICADOR

First published 2019 by Picador

This paperback edition first published 2022 by Picador
an imprint of Pan Macmillan
The Smithson, 6 Briset Street, London EC1M 5NR
EU representative: Macmillan Publishers Ireland Ltd, 1st Floor,
The Liffey Trust Centre, 117–126 Sheriff Street Upper,
Dublin 1, D01 YC43
Associated companies throughout the world
www.panmacmillan.com

ISBN 978-1-5290-3862-0

Copyright © Adam Kay 2019

The right of Adam Kay to be identified as the
author of this work has been asserted by him in accordance
with the Copyright, Designs and Patents Act 1988.

All rights reserved. No part of this publication may be reproduced,
stored in a retrieval system, or transmitted, in any form, or by any means
(electronic, mechanical, photocopying, recording or otherwise)
without the prior written permission of the publisher.

Pan Macmillan does not have any control over, or any responsibility for,
any author or third-party websites referred to in or on this book.

3 5 7 9 8 6 4 2

A CIP catalogue record for this book is available from the British Library.

Illustrations by Stephanie von Reiswitz

Typeset in Sabon by Palimpsest Book Production Ltd, Falkirk, Stirlingshire
Printed and bound by CPI Group (UK) Ltd, Croydon, CR0 4YY

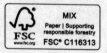

This book is sold subject to the condition that it shall not, by way of
trade or otherwise, be lent, hired out, or otherwise circulated without
the publisher's prior consent in any form of binding or cover other than
that in which it is published and without a similar condition including
this condition being imposed on the subsequent purchaser.

Visit www.picador.com to read more about all our books
and to buy them. You will also find features, author interviews and
news of any author events, and you can sign up for e-newsletters
so that you're always first to hear about our new releases.

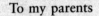

To my parents

(Not really to my parents, but they won't read beyond that page, and it's probably enough to get me back into the will.)

My publishers remain very keen that neither they nor I go to prison as a result of my books. To best achieve this, names, dates, personal information and clinical details have been changed. In my last book, I substituted all real names for the names of minor Harry Potter characters. This is not something I will be doing again.*

---

* This time they're all from *Home Alone*.

Contents

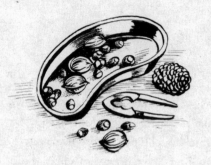

Introduction

Christmas is this pine-scented, tinsel-strewn timeout where, like it or not, everything just . . . stops. It's a temporary apocalypse where everyday norms are replaced with a fever dream of cheer and goodwill, and for an interminably long week, your daily grind goes out the window, replaced by weird, compulsory rituals.

You're forced into playing board games with your family, those blood-strangers you spend the rest of the year wilfully avoiding. You eat food like it's a competitive sport in which every kilo of meat or cheese gets you to the next level. And in order to cope with the steadily increasing strain of facetime with first-degree relatives, you don't so much flirt with alcoholism as fall into an S&M-heavy relationship with it.

It's a bizarro version of real life, an alternative reality where jollity is mandatory and apparently achieved only through a combination of charades, acid reflux, anger management and couch-sores. And all this is made possible because – thanks to the little baby Jesus – you no longer have to go to work. Well, *most* of you don't.

The NHS front line sadly doesn't get invited to Christ's all-you-can-eat birthday shindig. For medical personnel the world over, Christmas is just another day.

Coming but once a year – and thank fuck for that – the Yuletide brings more than its rightful share of hospital drama. Festive flus and pneumonia keep the respiratory teams busy, while norovirus and food poisoning are the season's special guest stars for the gastro doctors. Endocrinologists drag patients out of their mince-pie-induced diabetic comas, and the ortho-paedic wards heave with elderly patients who've gone full Jenga on the ice, shattering their hips like bags of biscuits.

A&E departments are busier than turkey farms, thanks to black eyes from carelessly popped cham-pagne corks, fleshy forearms seared by roasting tins, and children concussing themselves by hurtling down the stairs in the box their Scalextric came in. Not to mention the fairy-light electrocutions, turkey bones trapped in tracheas, and finger amputations from careless parsnip-chopping. Incidences of drunk driving go through the roof, often literally.

And then of course there's the carnage when families reach breaking point – usually some time between the Queen's speech and the late-night list shows. Under the influence of Christmas spirits and mistletoe, *crimes passionnels* erupt like violent genies in living rooms across the country, and still-sticky carving knives find their way into the nearest racist uncle.

I spent most of my medical career in obstetrics and gynaecology. Labouring mothers don't really have the option of staying home for a couple of days to 'see if it'll settle down' and, over in gynaecology, egged on by eggnog, there's a definite uptick in objects that have found themselves in orifices and are struggling with the return journey.

And then there's the heart-wrenching stuff. The middle-class pastime of Christmas Eve granny-dumping – bringing one's elderly or infirm relatives into hospital with some vague, fabricated medical complaint, so the dumpers can dedicate the next few days to solid partying, unfettered by caring for their parents.

Pushed to extremes by John Lewis adverts, Instagram exaggerators, and that terrible Paul McCartney song insisting that everyone else is simply having a wonderful Christmas time, many patients find this time of year too much to bear, and need to make use of our cruelly underfunded mental health services. And while of course there is never a good time to lose a loved one, there is something all the more harrowing about grief during the festive period, oppressively surrounded by global joy.

The annual winter health crisis rightly makes headlines every year, but over the festive period, the media – not wanting to piss in your Baileys – turns a blind eye, instead feeding us feel-good stories about a polar bear who's done a forward roll or some royal toddler trotting off to church in fur-trimmed couture. But, just as putting your hands over your eyes won't make you invisible, the patients don't go anywhere and the ambulances are still lined up outside A&E like lorries at Calais. And the staff are still there too, putting vocation over vacation. There's no reserve service, no fleet of Green Goddesses to give the healthcare professions a bit of time off. Instead, 1.4 million NHS employees divvy up the shifts and put in absurdly unsociable hours to ensure the rest of us make it through to the New Year in one piece.

Of the seven Christmas Days I was a practising doctor, I ended up on the wards for six of them. There were a few reasons for this, amounting to a perfect snowstorm. First of all, everyone thought I was Jewish, so assumed I wouldn't mind working on the least Jewish day of the year. In fairness to those people who thought I was Jewish, I *was* Jewish – and indeed still am – but with the emphasis very much on the 'ish'. I'm the kind of Jew who has a Christmas tree, doesn't go to synagogue, and in fact had to google the correct spelling of 'synagogue' when writing this sentence. Oh, and I don't believe in god, which I understand the more scrupulous practitioners generally do. Still, as far as my colleagues were concerned, I was certainly Jewish enough that I would happily sacrifice the annual twenty-four-hour TV-and-food-athon for the greater good.*

Added to this, I didn't – and indeed still don't – have any children. Christmas being a time for kids and all, the medics with young families would rise to the top of the Norway spruce and get the day off. I didn't begrudge them this, though for a while I did consider inventing some convenient yet imaginary offspring. The thankless toil of *actual* parenthood would probably have been an extremely expensive,

---

* Somehow my Jewish credentials didn't quite stretch to being able to skip work every Saturday. Talk about persecution.

stressful and inefficient way to get a free pass to eat sprouts on the same day as everyone else.

Due to the peripatetic nature of junior doctor training, I worked every Christmas in a different hospital, so I couldn't really call foul and complain I'd worked the previous year. That would be like refusing to buy the first round of drinks because you'd bought the last round the week earlier, for a completely different set of friends. In a pub 85 miles away.

Of course, I might have had more luck if I'd arranged the rota myself – the rota-organizers would always get a suspiciously easy set of shifts. But colour-coded spreadsheets were never my forte and the price the organizers paid for this privilege didn't seem worth the bother. I preferred to spend my already scant free time with my partner, not fielding angry calls from hard-done-by colleagues and wrestling with #VALUE! errors on Excel. Besides, even if you do end up avoiding Christmas Day, you'll almost certainly be stuck with the nightshift, or Boxing Day, or New Year's Eve. Hospitals attempt to slim down Christmas staffing to the bare minimum of doctors to provide safe care, but with 'bare minimum' generally representing the best-case scenario on a normal day, it's rather hard to tell the difference.

Ultimately, the shitty shifts still have to be filled and no one ever gets to avoid them all. There's about as much chance of a junior doctor getting the whole week off at Christmas as having enough cash to spend the time in Mustique, sipping vodka stingers across the pool from Bernie Ecclestone. Or Jeremy Hunt.

So here follow my diaries from those Christmases spent on the wards, removing babies and baubles from the various places they found themselves stuck.* But it wasn't all bad. At least I had an excuse not to spend time with my family.

* In my first book, *This is Going to Hurt*, the most common reasons for entries being omitted included 'too disgusting' or 'too Christmassy'. Here I make amends for both.

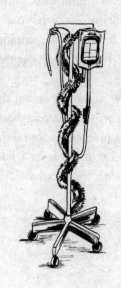

First Christmas

Twas the Christmas I had a urology job
Where bloke after bloke did weird shit to his knob

Monday, 20 December 2004

Patients generally have quite a few cards on their bedside tables and windowsills at this time of year, what with all the Get Well Soons and Merry Christmases.

Patient CG is recovering after a bowel resection, and his cubicle looks like a branch of Clintons.

On the ward round, my registrar Cliff chimes in with 'Someone's popular!' a millisecond too soon for me to lean in and whisper, 'Someone's wife just died . . .'*

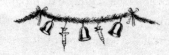

---

* Here are the medical ranks, and the corresponding level of servant as listed in Mrs Beeton's 1861 *Book of Household Management*:

House Officer – Scullery-maid/Stable boy
Senior House Officer – Maid/Groom
Registrar – Upper Housemaid/Footman
Senior Registrar – Housekeeper/House steward
Consultant – Master/Mistress of the house

At this stage I'm a house officer. According to Mrs B, the scullery-maid or stable boy would perform functions too menial or mucky for other members of the household – a fairly uncanny description of a house officer's role. Their annual salary was between £5 and £12 – again, not far off.

Wednesday, 22 December 2004

Sharing what I think is a top-level anecdote in the doctors' mess. I'm delighted with my story of the twenty-year-old guy whose half-arsed attempt at a costume for his Christmas party landed him in A&E.[*] It must have seemed a genius idea at the time, but he clearly didn't run it past anyone with common sense. He had wrapped his arms, legs, torso and head in layer upon layer of tinfoil, made a couple of holes for his eyes and one for his mouth, then dispatched himself to the party as a turkey. Several hours later, he collapsed, having desiccated himself to the human equivalent of a Ryvita, and requiring hospital admission for intravenous rehydration.

Disappointingly, no one is particularly impressed

---

[*] Fancy bloody dress. No one's heart has ever leapt at that particular line on the party invite – you'll end up either being the only person who's dressed up or the only person who hasn't. Or you'll pitch it colossally wrong, spunking an entire morning and two hundred quid in the National Theatre hire shop while every other guest has dug out some devil horns or a cardboard Prince Charles mask. And how the fuck is anyone meant to take a shit while dressed as Spider-Man?

by my turkey tale.* One of the Senior House Officers, Frank, tries to salvage it for me: 'Had he also crammed two kilos of stuffing up his arse?' Alas not.

Frank counters with the story of a similar patient he had last year, who decided to cover every surface of his skin with gaffer tape. 'Wasn't for a party though . . .' he adds.

I ask why, then remember why most people do most things, and thus find myself introduced – at the tender age of twenty-four – to the sexual kink of mummification.

Not much has changed in the three millennia since the process was pioneered by Ramesses and his pals, though these days people leave a couple of nostril holes for breathing. (And a third, rather larger hole on the reverse side.) Though, as this patient discovered, gaffer tape has its limitations as a mummification material. Upon 'emergence', as is apparently the term for unwrapping, it not only exfoliates effectively but also does a pretty thorough job of removing all body hair. Oh, and it circumcises.

---

* Doctors are a tough crowd at the best of times, and stories of patient idiocy are a bit like antibiotics: they lose their power in a population overexposed to them.

Saturday, 25 December 2004

So here it is, Merry Christmas, everybody's having fun. Somewhere else. I'm ringing in my first 25th December on the wards by doing an impression of a smiley doctor off the telly, but it grates any time a patient or colleague wishes me a happy Christmas.

I'm trying to forget what I'm missing and treat it like a normal day, but every few minutes there's a fresh reminder. Decorations hang limply around each corner, looking like they've come out of the same box every year since word came from Bethlehem about this exciting new festival. My phone pulsates with jolly seasonal text messages, like I've got a malfunctioning dildo in my pocket.

Santa might be putting his feet up after a long night, but his pal the Grim Reaper never gets the day off. And so I find myself sitting in a side room with a distressed family, having The Chat about mum/gran. They know the punchline before I even start the story – a doctor is never going to summon an extended family to sit on uncomfortable chairs at short notice on Christmas Day to tell them they've won fifty grand on a scratch card.

Granny is outnumbered by E. coli bacteria in her bloodstream to the tune of several billion to one, and there's now only one way this can end. It doesn't prevent her family holding out for a final dramatic plot twist.

'There must be more you can try,' begs a distraught son. Honestly, if there was, I'd have already tried it to avoid discussions like this. Bad news is never easy to hear, but it's never easy to deliver either. Drawn faces, with sad, set mouths; eyes already dull and resigned; hands clenched together, knuckles straining at the skin. Some will sob, some will scream, some will just stare blankly into the abyss I've created. Here goes another one.

With every fibre of my calm and professionalism, I explain that, even though she's been a fighter throughout, her organs have started to fail and she's deteriorating fast, despite the fluids and antibiotics we've been giving her. As their eyes well up, I tell them that we've already asked the ITU doctors to review her and they agreed it wouldn't be kind to pursue aggressive treatment that would ultimately have no chance of working.

Hoping to show empathy through my body language, I lean in to say all we can do now is keep her comfortable and concentrate on her dignity. As I do so, I inadvertently lean on my tie.

It's a seasonal tie – a deep, night-sky blue with dear old Santa on his sleigh perched right up near the knot. Moving down the tie we come to Prancer and Dancer and the rest of the reindeer massive, with Rudolph proudly front and centre. Crucially, and disastrously, underneath Rudolph's red nose – and now the pressure of my elbow – is a button that activates a tinny speaker to blast out a frantic MIDI rendition of 'Jingle Bells'.

I turn ketchup red, apologize and jab at my abdomen. But all I succeed in doing is restarting the fucking tune. After half a dozen failed attempts to silence it, over the course of what feels like fifteen years, I run outside and hurl the tie onto the nursing station.

As I head back into the room, thinking of superlatives to add to my apologies, one of the daughters is in the middle of an uncontrollable laughing fit and everyone else is smiling. Maybe there *is* an easier way to deliver bad news, after all.

It's 5 p.m. before I manage my Christmas dinner (stolen toast from the ward kitchen, served with low-ranking Quality Streets), and I'm hit by the sinking realization that I'm not even looking forward to going home – I'll be trudging back to an empty flat. H* is off doing familial duties and my own nearest and dearest are either not particularly near or not particularly dear. Anyway, the odds of actually finishing at 8 p.m. are lower than a salamander's scrotum, so at least there'll only be ninety minutes of actual Christmas Day to spend at home by myself.

Duncan, one of the other house officers, comes into the kitchen brandishing a bleak-looking cracker he's found. We pull it, then roll our eyes at the homeopathically weak joke. He heads back to the ward in his paper hat and I stand by the microwave, taking the fortune-telling magic fish out of its wrapper. Its head rolls up in my palm, and I consult the legend for its psychic take. 'Moving head: Jealousy'.

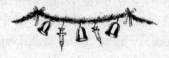

---

* H was my partner at that time. ('At that time' – yeah, sorry for the spoiler if you haven't read my first book.)

Sunday, 26 December 2004

Full marks to the anaesthetist wearing a badge that says: 'He sees you when you're sleeping, he knows when you're awake'.

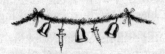

Monday, 27 December 2004

A lot of the reward for this job comes in the form of a warm glow. It doesn't make you look any less tired, you can't pay the rent with it, and it's worth a lot less than the social life you've traded it for, but this comforting aura of goodness and purpose definitely throws light into some dark corners and helps you withstand a lot of the shit.

The Force is strongest when working over Christmas. This year I have donated Christmas Day, Boxing Day and today to the NHS, so my glow can be seen and felt from the outer reaches of Canis Major. But it's about to be eclipsed and extinguished by the actions of a literal saint.

I get a bleep from switchboard at 2 p.m. It's Kate,

one of the SHOs, asking me to meet her down in reception. I harrumph my way down – *I'm busy up here . . . what does she want . . . she's not even working today.*

When I get there she's smiling warmly, like Princess Diana at an orphanage. She sticks her hand out and asks for my bleep. 'My husband's taking the kids to the park – why don't you go out for a few hours?' My brain can't process this level of unexpected and extreme altruism. At first I can't understand if she's asking me to babysit the children or go dogging with her husband, but when the penny drops and I realize I'm being invited to play hookey, I manage to stutter out some vague vowel sounds by way of thanks. I hand over the bleep slowly, like it's a grenade, just in case this is a trick. But, no, off she skips to the ward with it.

I wander down the high street feeling bewildered, like I've had a phone call telling me I'm now the king or have found an amulet that gives me the ability to fly.

I stop off for a coffee then mooch across to the cinema. My options are an action film I quite want to see but have missed the first half of, a family blockbuster I don't especially want to see, or something arty and French that I would rather boil my eyes in molten manure than watch. I choose the least-worst option and settle down for 120 minutes of Pixar.

The film is actually much better than I thought it would be, and I even get to have my guilty-pleasure treat – something I only eat in darkness and either alone or in the company of people who've known me over two decades and on whom I have plenty of reciprocal blackmail material – a tub of sweet popcorn with a large bag of Skittles mixed in. All for only slightly more than the price of a week in Santorini!

I return to work, high on e-numbers and the kindness of the human spirit.

'Did you get up to anything nice?' asks Kate.

'Yes actually,' I beam back. 'I went to see *The Incredibles*.'

'Oh, that's so sweet you call them that! Do they live round here?'

Did I come out the wrong exit of the cinema and emerge into a parallel universe?

'It's sweet?'

'Yes, that you call your parents The Incredibles!'

I smile like the wonderful, benevolent son I am not, and tell her that, yes, I do. That way, she can at least think she did a nice thing for an equally nice person – not a bastard who never even considered seeing his family and instead just went to the cinema and got off his tits on additives.

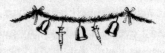

Wednesday, 29 December 2004

'Help me out here,' I say to the patient after I finally tire of our silent staring contest. 'Have you got *any* idea at all what might have caused it?'

The twenty-year-old stays mute, only shrugging his shoulders and brushing his hair out of his eyes as I examine his translucent-skinned penis: a canapé-sized recreation of the bag of giblets you used to find inside supermarket chickens.

I don't want to accuse him of dipping it in a pot of acid every evening, but that's pretty much what it looks like. Whatever he's been doing, he's managed to wear away his foreskin to such a watery shine that I certainly won't be ordering summer rolls next time I'm in a Vietnamese restaurant.

Twenty minutes later we've all learned something. I've learned what kind of person clicks on penis enlargement adverts on the internet and parts with actual money for magic cock-growing cream. He's learned the cream he'd pinned his hopes on is almost certainly a potent steroid, and that steroids thin the skin. And, unless of course the wretched thing started out the size of a drawing pin, it unfortunately hasn't had the desired effect.

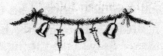

Thursday, 30 December 2004

Patient VY is eighty-two years old and was admitted last week with a strangulated hernia,* requiring emergency surgery. I suspect he's keen to go home, given he's sat up in a chair and dressed like Mr Banks from *Mary Poppins* in a three-piece suit with matching tie and handkerchief. All that's missing is a pocket watch. I jokily say how nice it is that he's made the effort for my ward round.

---

* A hernia is when a bit of your bowel (usually) pokes through a weak point in muscles or other tissues. A strangulated hernia is an emergency that occurs if the bowel's blood supply gets cut off, generally causing vomiting and the kind of pain you'd expect if your intestines were in a vice.

'See?' he tells his daughter, who is sitting next to him. She rolls her eyes and explains that the ambulance had to wait for five minutes while her dad changed into formal wear, despite the eye-watering agony he must have been in. 'No excuse to look slovenly,' he tells me.

'And then,' she adds, 'he wouldn't let them take him to hospital until he'd brushed his teeth!'

'In case I needed mouth-to-mouth,' he explains.

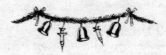

Friday, 31 December 2004

I can smell it before I arrive on the ward, the unmistakable pong of bleach and obsequiousness. One of our beloved health ministers will be visiting today.*

---

* In an example of 'don't know what you've got till it's gone' that would make Joni Mitchell urgently rewrite 'Big Yellow Taxi', I worked as a doctor under Labour governments, before politicians of the other persuasion started hacking back health budgets like they were overgrown wisteria. Since I was a kid, every time Satan's merry-go-round span another rotation and gave us a new Health Secretary, I would ask my dad – a

These cartoon villains must travel the length of the country, thinking the entire UK smells like Flash All-Purpose Cleaner.

No doubt he'll parrot whichever plaudit he's written on the back of his hand. 'Thank you for working so hard' will probably feature – though presumably any job looks like hard work when yours only occupies 150 days of the year and involves falling asleep on leather benches and eating taxpayer-subsidized beef Wellington.

And like the tree that falls in the forest, if the minister isn't accompanied by a phalanx of press and photographers, would he even be here at all? I conjure up the carefully framed photograph in tomorrow's papers: the minister pretending to look interested and angling his bald spot away from the camera while exchanging pleasantries with a nurse. The nurse will somehow manage to resist all her natural urges and smile back at him rather than spiking him in the neck with a scalpel. Some tinsel will be artfully

---

GP – what the new boss was going to be like. His answer was always the same: 'They'll be the worst one since the last one.' This generally proved right. Personally I think of Health Secretaries like Defence Against the Dark Arts teachers in the *Harry Potter* books. They're obviously going to turn out to be evil, but you'll have to wait a while to find out precisely how.

draped on the wall to remind us that not only health-care staff but, much more importantly, politicians are working hard over the festive period.

I suspect I won't be one of the chosen few to shake the dead, clammy hand of one of the government's weasels-in-chief (would it snap off at the wrist?), but I still find myself worrying about my duty to the patients' confidentiality. It would be unforgivable if any identifying information were photographed and published, so I dash over to the ward whiteboard. The names of all patients are initialized in any case, but who can say if that's enough of a cipher to adequately protect their anonymity? Ever-diligent, I err toward caution and put them under even deeper cover, replacing the initials of the eight patients in the first bay with some totally random letters that just happened to come into my head.

F.U.

C.K.

Y.O.

U.T.

O.N.

Y.B.

L.A.

I.R.

Tuesday, 4 January 2005

It's important to have a hobby, I suppose. A way of switching your brain into a different gear and shaking out the stresses that have been clogging up your neurons after a hard day's work. I've got writing and playing the piano, which are, if not enough, then all I've got the time for. For other people it's jogging, or macramé, or track days, or fishing. And for Patient AM – a hip-hop artist in his twenties – it's visiting prostitutes and handing over a wad of cash in return for having them stick needles through his penis. Acupuncture as reimagined by the Marquis de Sade.

But you know how it is over Christmas – everyone's on their holidays, so you have to make do with a temp. You go to the barber and your normal guy's away, so your hair doesn't sit quite right. The Christmas postman doesn't know to leave your parcels behind the wheelie bin if you're out, so they end up at some godforsaken depot 30 miles away. And the locum prostitute uses a different bore of needle when she's driving them through your cock, which explains Patient AM's referral from A&E to urology with 'difficulty passing urine'. And not in the normal sense of painful or poor flow. Quite the opposite in fact – it was more a case of controlling it. In Eminemmental's own words, he's got a 'cock like a colander'. I insert an (advent) catheter, admit him to the ward, and resist the temptation to text about thirty people.*

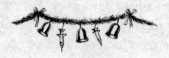

---

* Although admittedly, I have just published his story in a book.

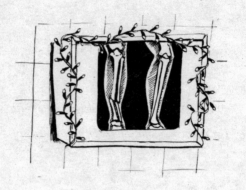

Second Christmas

While Santa is flying his sleigh full of gifts
I'm wrenching out babies on unending shifts

Friday, 16 December 2005

I put the Sonicaid probe onto a mum's abdomen in antenatal clinic and turn it on, waiting for the familiar *SWOOSH SWOOSH SWOOSH* of baby's heartbeat. Nothing. Bloody batteries. I flick the on/off switch a couple more times, then apologize to the patient.

'Sorry, I think this one's dead.'

As the mum's face collapses like a bouncy castle at closing time, I urgently clarify: 'The Sonicaid! The Sonicaid!'

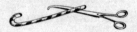

Tuesday, 20 December 2005

Christmas card from Mr Polinksi, one of the consultants:

Wishing you and yours
a happy and healthy Christmas
and all the best for 2006.

Dictated but not signed to avoid delay.

Wednesday, 21 December 2005

It started with a length of tinsel being Blu-tacked to the gynaecology ward wall in the shape of an ECG trace.* Then the Christmas tree was decorated with a bunch of inflated rubber gloves and a few baubles fashioned from ring pessaries. The gynae nurses pimped a few speculums with googly eyes and red cardboard noses to turn them into the world's most repulsive reindeer – you would not want these lads guiding your sleigh *anywhere* tonight.

This evening I made a beautiful wreath with the help of one of the healthcare assistants. We took a box of out-of-date condoms, unwrapped and unfurled them, braided them into a big circle and stuck it on

---

* I never quite know where to draw the line with explaining terminology. All the words make sense to *me* – whether it's haemoptysis (hacking up blood) or hospital (the sprawling, dilapidated building in which you hack up said blood). Anyway, an ECG, or electrocardiogram, is the squiggly printout of your heart's electrical activity, much beloved of medical drama title sequences. It's obtained by putting sticky pads on your chest, arms and legs. For good electrical contact, men often need their chests shaved first. I once asked a medical student to shave a patient before an ECG. Fuck knows what the poor patient thought was happening when the student came into his cubicle, removed his five o'clock shadow and tidied up his sideburns.

the door to the ward. Sadly, it didn't see out a whole shift before some Scrooge pulled it down.

Thankfully they're yet to spot that the fairy sitting on top of the tree has an umbilical cord knitted from suture material, dangling menacingly from under her tutu.

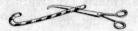

Saturday, 24 December 2005

Trying to work out whether I'm hallucinating through lack of food or lack of rest, but no, it seems *everyone* can hear a brass band playing 'O Little Town of Bethlehem'. It's an A for effort but a JESUS CHRIST NO PLEASE STOP for quality. When I'm done with my needlework, restoring a perineum back to factory settings, I go and investigate, wandering to the second-floor railings and leaning over to identify the source of this hell-scream. In the foyer are about six or seven schoolkids with instruments and a choir of about thirty more, standing around them in a semicircle.

As they honk and wail their way through the

classics, decreasing in confidence with each verse, I find myself inexplicably . . . what is this feeling? Not quite enjoying it, but . . . OK, fine, enjoying it. It's like this cacophony is somehow magically tapping into happy memories of Christmases gone by and giving my limbic system a hug.

Seeing these kids dressed up smartly in their uniforms on Christmas Eve (when I'm sure they'd much rather be giving their presents exploratory rattles or learning the basics of gang violence) – well, it's like the end of a Richard Curtis movie.

My bleep goes off and I feel strangely reluctant to head back to labour ward. A man walks past me, leans over the railings and says to his partner, 'Good advert for contraception.' I'm about to tut pointedly when a patient from yesterday gestures at me and says, 'You should try having this bloke rip you a new one.'

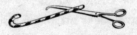

Sunday, 25 December 2005

It's my first Christmas on labour ward. I've been trying to convince myself (and H, with more limited success) that doing two years on the trot means being off work for the big day next year is practically a certainty.

Thankfully, it's jolly enough on labour ward, and there's a decent haul of festive names. Welcome to baby Holly and baby Casper, though in full disclosure, Lesley – a midwife in her sixties – had to explain why Casper was at all Christmassy. I just assumed it was one of those names that normal people give their dogs or upper-class people call their eighth son. But it turns out I nodded off in RE one too many times and the names of the three wise men had passed me by until today. At least the kid's not called Balthazar, limiting his career options to society photographer or Disney baddie.

Casper's arrival kicks off a long discussion among the midwives of various other festive first names – from Robin to Grace to Gabriel, then talk of the ones that have fallen out of fashion – the Carols and the Glorias. Lesley looks wistful: 'Noel always used to be very popular. But Edmonds seems to have fucked that.'

We're interrupted by my bleep. Patient BK is thirty weeks pregnant and bleeding from her left earlobe. To be more accurate, blood is cascading out of her left earlobe. Between what's soaked through the tea towels she brought in, the clothes she's wearing and the scrubs I'm wearing, I think it must be a litre. I don't know what's happening, but I do at least know that blood is a finite resource.

I call Stan, one of the registrars. If 'first do no harm' tops the list of medical commandments, then 'don't blag it' can't be that far down.* He suspects I'm being a drama queen and my patient just has a spot on her ear. 'It's not a *litre* – a little blood goes a very long way.' I beg him to come quickly, then put in a drip, send some bloods off, order four units of crossmatched blood, and hold some large swabs very hard against her ear.

Stan arrives a few minutes later. 'Wow, yes, that's definitely a litre.' And counting. He asks the same questions I did: 'Has this happened before?' – no.

* I was surprised to discover quite early on in this job that patients don't care in the slightest when you hold up your hands and tell them you're going to call in someone more senior. They actually seem to like it – they're getting to see someone better. It's an unexpected upgrade at check-in, a double-yolker.

'Do you have any blood clotting disorders?' – no. 'Have you hurt your ear?' – no. He performs a brief but puzzled examination of the patient, although there's not much to see beyond the jet of blood. He then does his own phone-a-friend. Mr Hess, the labour ward consultant, advises him to give the patient a shot of steroids to help the baby's lungs in case it needs premature delivery today, and to call the Ear, Nose and Throat team.

A general surgical registrar answers the bleep because ENT are on call from home today.* He takes a look at the patient – who is, understandably, looking pretty worried by this point – and tells the ENT registrar she needs to come in. It's all become rather more serious now – a parade of increasingly specialized doctors but no hint of a solution. The patient is moved to the high dependency unit on labour ward, and a further four units of blood are on their way. The ENT registrar drags her consultant in from home immediately, and the rest of us feel better about not knowing the answer ourselves.

The ENT consultant tells the patient he needs to

_____

* ENT is commonly known as Early Nights and Tennis – a good choice of specialty if you like a quiet Christmas. See also, dermaholiday.

operate immediately to stop the bleeding and seems to have some kind of plan as to how to achieve this. Mr Hess comes in. With every passing minute more people arrive – anaesthetists, interventional radiologists, haematologists. A matryoshka of medics.

But labour ward never stops, and as I can't claim to be bringing much to this particular party, I head off to review the nine patients who have accumulated in triage while we've been playing 'What The Fuck Is Happening To This Patient And If She Dies Is It My Fault?' Then it's down to A&E for some gynae goings-on before running upstairs to assist in a caesarean.

By the time I come up for air, I hear that Patient BK is out of theatre, baby still in situ and doing well, and there's no more spurting blood. The diagnosis was an AV malformation in her ear.* Not something I've ever read about before, but 'bodies don't read textbooks', as the *bon mot* goes. They clearly don't read calendars either. Between the doctors, nurses, midwives and theatre staff, she must have had twenty

---

* An AV (arteriovenous) malformation is a rare manufacturing fault where a spaghetti junction of arteries and veins forms. They most commonly occur in the brain, but can pop up anywhere. They have a tendency to bleed heavily, and this happens more frequently in pregnancy.

people looking after her, many of them hauled away from their families halfway through Christmas dinner. Life goes on – and that can be negative as well as positive – whether it's Christmas Day, New Year's Eve or Albatross Appreciation Day.

I realize with a shudder that I haven't had time to look at my phone since all this started. There are at least a dozen messages from H, whose good humour leaks away with each subsequent one until 'Appreciate you're busy – won't interrupt you any more.'

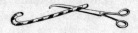

Saturday, 31 December 2005

'Say that again?' asked Mitch.

'She's got extremely heavy thrush, with green and red flecks in it,' I say.

'So, blood then?'

'No, it's not blood, it's . . . shiny. Like bits of toenail polish.'

'Is it bits of toenail polish?'

'I don't think so . . .'

I'm about to have another go at explaining but

Mitch stops me, holding his finger aloft as if he's about to conduct an orchestra, then walks off to review the patient. He glides back five minutes later, looking like he's worked out the plot to *Donnie Darko*.

'You didn't ask the right questions,' he says, every syllable a dunce's cap thudding onto my head. 'You see, 99 per cent of the time you'll get the answer by taking a thorough history, before you even lay a hand on the patient.'

I know I have to let his pompous little speech burn out before interrupting. Registrars like to do this kind of thing now and again to show they've 'still got it', like your uncle squeezing himself into his Speedos despite the gasps of terrified onlookers around the hotel pool. Once he's done, I ask what the right question was.

'Have you recently been using a candy cane as a dildo?'

Of course! I'll add that to my list of icebreakers.

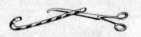

39

Sunday, 1 January 2006

When the posters announced that the hospital was getting new discharge summary* software for 2006, like the world's most boring New Year's Resolution, I don't think any of us imagined the big changeover would happen within the final echoes of Big Ben's last bong on the first of January. To give the hospital an unusual amount of credit, they've laid on a bunch of IT 'helpers', wandering the corridors wearing bright sashes like regional semi-finalists in a Slimmer of the Year competition. The bloke assigned to the gynaecology ward agreed that the timing left a little to be desired. 'At least we're on triple pay!' he trilled, hitting keys on a computer like a lab rat nudging the trapdoor for a treat. Triple pay? *You* may be but *we* certainly are not. I hope he spends the spoils on Aquafresh – his halitosis practically phones ahead to tell you it's coming.

I guess we should be grateful our technology is being coerced, if not into the twenty-first century,

---

* For once, a term that's less revolting than you might fear. A discharge summary is the paperwork that gives the patient and their GP a potted history of their hospital stay, the medication they're going home with, and any planned follow-up.

then certainly the mid-to-late twentieth. The old system was the stuff of Bob Cratchit's nightmares: the doctor would write a summary of the patient's stay on triplicate carbon paper. The top copy was for the notes, the middle one for the patient, and the bottom copy – with its faint suggestion of the original writing (unless you get a doctor prepared to channel all his anger into a biro) – posted off to the patient's GP. But from today, all the information goes straight onto the computer system . . . before a copy is printed off and – give me strength – *faxed* to the GP.

Technology may change, but the patients certainly don't. On this morning's ward round I meet Patient AW, who saw in the new year with a bang. Followed by a whimper.

Finding herself in a suitor's bedroom, in need of some vaginal lubrication, and having found no joy in either the bedside table or bathroom cabinet, she went to the kitchen for inspiration and returned with a tub of peanut butter. While she should definitely have carried on rooting through the cupboards, peanut butter wasn't the most terrible choice – it's an oil-based spread, plus it offers the option of smooth or crunchy, for your added 'pleasure'. Downsides include the fact that oil-based lubricants are kryptonite to condoms, not to mention the potential for extreme mess: no cleaner is going to believe the brown slick on the sheet is peanut butter. Also, some people have peanut allergies. Patient AW, for example.

'But . . . whyyyy?' I asked, stretching the word longer than Annie Lennox ever managed.

'I assumed it was only a problem, you know, up the other end,' she explained. I imagine she was too caught up in the moment to google it, but her theory proved incorrect. Luckily, she escaped the worst-case scenario of breathing difficulties and ultimately, well, not breathing at all, but she did develop vaginal and vulval swelling to the extent she couldn't pass urine. My colleagues on the nightshift had catheterized her, washed everything out (making them the automatic winners of any 'who had the worst New Year's Eve?' conversation) and started her on steroids and anti-histamines.

This morning the disaster zone has calmed down, the catheter has been removed and she's peeing successfully without it, so I discharge her home. We're in mutual agreement she shouldn't engage in future use of intravaginal Sun-Pat.

And so to try out the new computer system. The IT helper – cheese, onion, and sewage sandwich for lunch, it appears – is talking me through the software.

Apparently I need to choose the diagnosis from a telephone directory of pre-programmed, ultra-specific options.

'How would you describe the patient's diagnosis in one or two words?' he asks.

I pause. 'Vaginaphylaxis?'

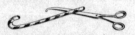

Wednesday, 4 January 2006

After a couple of months of waiting on the edge of my seat, the final adjudication is through on the locum nightshift I did in October, when the clocks went back and I put in a timesheet for thirteen hours.

'Shifts are defined as twelve hours,' the email barks, 'irrespective of the number of hours worked.' Who needs the scientific laws of space and time when you've got whichever handbook this bastard flicked through to get the answer? I'm pretty sure that if I'd worked the night the clocks went forward, I'd only get paid for eleven.

'I don't want to die,' Patient JM said, plaintively. None of us want to die, of course – it's human nature – but I was surprised to hear it from the mouth of a ninety-one-year-old. We're conditioned to describe this as a good innings, but when you're lying in a hospital bed with all signs pointing towards your permanent exit from the planet, age doesn't really come into it. If anything, those extra couple of decades thinking about the final page of the story probably make it all the more difficult to approach.

I decided the best thing to do was pretend I hadn't heard what she'd said, and continued to insert the drip in her hand, as if I was concentrating so hard it had rendered me deaf. She waited until the drip was in, then touched my hand, her skin so loose it didn't feel quite human. 'Is this it?' she asked, her eyes searching mine as I stared back vacantly. 'Am I dying?'

She knew. I'd given her tacit confirmation by not answering the first time. And she *was* dying – it wouldn't be more than a day away. The more patients I see, the more I can tell – it's not just the black-and-white of measurable things like respiratory rates and full blood counts, or even the clinical signs like laboured breathing and mottled skin. It's an aura, if doctors are allowed to use such a word, and working in gynae oncology has made me far more attuned to it.

I'd never been asked this before, and I had no idea how to deal with it. Every day brings new challenges I don't have the cheat sheet for, like a recurring nightmare where you turn up for your finals drunk and unprepared.

After too long a pause, I copped out and lied: 'No, don't be silly!' Not just 'No' but 'No, don't be silly!' – negating her, throwing her off the scent, in reply to the bravest question of all. She looked back at me without a hint of relief and pretended to accept my answer with a faint smile, then slowly leaned her head back to look up at the ceiling, as if imagining herself among the stars. Once eye contact was broken, I made my excuses and scuttled off.*

I realize I never actually talk about death with patients – their families, my colleagues, sure, but not them. For the rest of the nightshift, I obsess over

---

* The eminent palliative care doctor Kathryn Mannix writes beautifully and powerfully about this topic in her book, *With the End in Mind*. Not just healthcare professionals, but all of us need to be honest and unafraid to talk about death.

what I should have said. All she wanted was someone to be straight with her and confirm what she knew deep down. At ninety-one she's earned that right. Instead, I was too scared to tell the truth, and I let her down.

When that day arrives for me, if I'm able to ask my doctor that question, I want them to be honest – and then I want them to hook me up to the largest bottle of vodka they can carry.

At the end of the shift, I trudge back to her ward. I tell myself I'm going to speak to her again, giving myself a motivational pep talk as I go. You've got this, I say, you owe it to her. But, shamefully, I'm half hoping that I won't have to.

There's an empty bed in bay three. I don't have to.

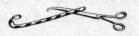

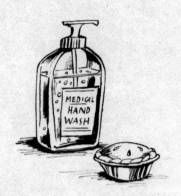

Third Christmas

Come Dancer! Come Prancer! Come Rudolph! Come Comet!
Come rescue me now cos I'm covered in vomit

Monday, 20 November 2006

The Christmas rota has been emailed round and – jingle balls – I've drawn the short straw.

Colleagues give me sympathetic looks all day. Donald, one of the other SHOs, pats me on the back. 'Hard lines, mate.' I open my mouth to tell him it's fine, when he jumps straight in with, 'My mum's dying and it's the last Christmas I'm going to spend with her.'

'Oh god, Don – I'm so sorry, I had no idea. I wasn't asking to swap . . .'

'No no, it's my suggestion for you – email them back with *that* as your excuse.'

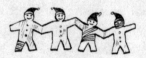

Tuesday, 19 December 2006

We're invited to donate a fiver to charity and wear Christmassy clothes today. Most people have gone for jaunty jumpers, so the air crackles with acrylic charge, staff becoming human Van de Graaff generators if they get within a foot of each other. I've cracked out my musical Rudolph tie, representing as it does the sole contents of my Christmas wardrobe.

We set off on the gynae ward round. I clasp my hands together a few inches away from my chest to stop anyone or anything bashing into my tie and setting off a chorus or twelve of 'Jingle Bells'. Even though I look like some mad medical Buddha, it's not me who attracts attention.

'I'm very sorry to ask this,' Marv, one of the registrars, says to Miss Balzak. 'Those reindeer on your jumper – do you think they might be . . . having a bit of "ladies and gentlemen"?'

Miss Balzak looks down at her sweater: racing green with white cross-stitched rows of snowflakes top and bottom and three reindeer in between. The middle reindeer is subtly, but quite unmistakably, mounting the reindeer on the right and being rimmed by the smaller reindeer on the left. Not the usual look you'd expect on someone who makes Miss Marple look like Sharon Stone.

'Oh, for goodness' sake,' says Miss Balzak. 'They bloody are, aren't they?' She'd picked it up from a stall in Camden Market when she was out Christmas shopping because she thought it looked fun, not quite noticing just how much fun Rudolph's red nose was having.

'Shall we wait while you change?' asks Marv.

Miss Balzak ignores him. 'Who's next? Bay eight?'

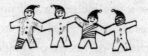

Friday, 22 December 2006

Patient FJ is pushing, I'm on forceps duty, and the radio is shitting out the Christmas classics. I've done my second pull (accompanied by Johnny Mathis), the baby is nearly out, and we're all catching our breaths before the grand finale.

The patient suddenly shouts at the radio.

'No, Johnny. That is *not* what happens when a child is born.'

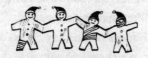

Saturday, 23 December 2006

As crap as it is working in hospital over Christmas, it's easy to forget how much worse it must be for the patients, so it's all hands on deck over the next couple of days to get anyone home who's vaguely well enough to wheel or drag themselves off the ward. Patients are Lazarus-ed out of their beds and switched from festive-sounding IV antibiotics to the more portable oral variety, to get them back to the bosom of their loving families. The added bonus being that, with the indentation from the hospital wristband still on their arm, they'll be excused so much as pouring themselves an Advocaat, let alone carving the turkey, mopping the floor or consoling a child who wanted an Xbox but got an atlas.

Patient BC is seventy-two and well enough post-op to go home. I've quite enjoyed springing from bedside to bedside breaking good news, like a game-show host telling a contestant they've won a Mini Metro or a luxury holiday for four to Torremolinos. But when I get to Patient BC, her face doesn't light up like the others – she just mutters 'OK' and looks away.

I hover.

'Hmm. Your wound is looking a bit red, though,'

I offer. It isn't. She looks back round at me. 'Maybe we should keep an eye on it over the next few days?'

Her entire body relaxes. It's the kind of reaction you only usually see when you tell a patient their biopsy result is normal. I daren't ask what kind of desperate domestic set-up, or lack thereof, means she'd rather be here than at home, but at least we can offer her a roof, a bit of company and some NHS parsnips. It's a new twist on the classic 'granny dump', but I suspect this is actually the biggest help I've been to a patient all day.

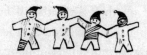

Sunday, 24 December 2006

'Spot diagnosis?' asks one of the paediatric SHOs, showing a photo on his phone around the doctors' mess. It's a child aged about four with a green face. Not 'a bit peaky' green, but 'uranium in the sandpit' luminescent. Maybe his dad's the Incredible Hulk and he's having his first tantrum?

Answer: he'd dismantled his mum's novelty earrings and shoved an LED up his nose, not realizing how much better a red light would have been for a Christmas anecdote.

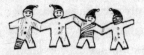

Monday, 25 December 2006

Despite all my best efforts, it's a hat-trick: three Christmases on the trot opening up patients instead of presents. Tentative efforts to swap with colleagues were batted away like bluebottles. Not sure what I expected them to say. 'Bollocks to my husband, angelic children, and plans that have been set in stone for months – sure, I'll spend the day knee-deep in amniotic fluid instead.'

H took the news pretty well, all things considered, but I'm still half-expecting to find every pair of shoes I own filled with cranberry sauce when I get home.

Cheerier relationship news with the discovery that Molly, one of the midwives, is dating Petr, an A&E nurse. It's like when you hear that a pair of celebrities have coupled up and you try to imagine them together – cooking pasta, doing the big shop, arguing, fucking, reverse parking, watching *Corrie* –

before giving them the Gladiator-style thumbs-up or thumbs-down.

It's been going on for months apparently, but they've never broadcast the fact. We only found out because they're both working today and Petr has rocked up on labour ward to surprise Molly with a full Christmas dinner for two: lovingly prepared last night, transported in Tupperware and now spinning round in the labour ward microwave. He even colluded with Sondra, the midwife supervisor, who has given Molly a break and cleared the rest of us out of the coffee room so they can have some time together. Sondra has even laid on a tablecloth (well, blue drape) for that extra touch of class.

The rest of us walk up and down the corridor a few times more than might be strictly necessary so we can steal a peek through the coffee room door. On the face of it, this is not a Christmas dinner that will be troubling the Michelin guide any time soon – nuked roast potatoes, desiccated turkey and coagulated gravy wolfed down in a thirty-minute lunch break in a room that should probably be condemned. But it's the thought behind it – the rom-com sweetness – that elevates it to the most beautiful thing I have seen all week, and makes me physically jealous of a Christmas spent together.

I'm bleeped away to see Patient NW, who has come to labour ward with reduced fetal movements at thirty-eight weeks.* The CTG† is a bit manky and the baby's breech – so caesarean section it is. 'Oh, for fuck's sake,' she says.

I reassure her everything's going to be absolutely fine for her and baby. 'Oh, it's not that,' she groans. 'My other one was born on Christmas Day too. Everyone's going to think I do this deliberately to save on presents.'

I leave the room and see Petr and Molly snatching

---

* Mums know when there's something wrong with their unborn children. They're connected by more than just an umbilical cord, it's an almost psychic bond, and it's a negligent obstetrician who disregards a mother's hunch. This is, of course, in stark contrast to almost every other branch of medicine, where the mad shit that's resulted from a patient's frantic googling carries a roughly zero per cent chance of tallying up with their actual diagnosis.

Sometimes reduced fetal movements are a sign of something being wrong, but often a baby has simply decided that they're 'doing downtime' – an exciting glimpse into their future teenage aesthetic – and soon comes round when mum drinks a glass of cold water. It's the maternofetal version of chucking a bucket of water over their head. Again, worth remembering for their teenage years.

† CTG – or cardiotocograph – is a recording of baby's heart rate and mum's contractions that continually streams out of a printer like ticker tape in 1950s Wall Street.

a kiss before they shoot off for another seven hours of the great British public's contusions and contractions. Thumbs-up from me. Not sure I want to imagine them fucking, though.

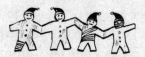

Wednesday, 27 December 2006

A patient's ten-year-old son has been sitting wordlessly for an hour in triage while his mum waits to be seen, staring at his laptop screen and tapping away. A Christmas present, I assume. It makes an irritating beeping sound every second or two. I should confiscate it and donate it to the nursing station – it looks twenty times newer and more advanced than any computer I've seen in the hospital, like comparing the Hubble telescope with a £1.99 pair of tartan-framed novelty glasses from a whisky distillery gift shop.

Beep. Beep. Beep. Still, at least it's not a drum kit. His mum notices I'm staring and smiles, under the misapprehension that I think her son is in any way sweet.

'He's really into his codeine,' she tells me. Jesus Christ. Hours of phone calls to child protection officers flash before my eyes, jackknifing across the rest of my shift. She looks at my clearly troubled face and repeats: 'He's really into his coding.'

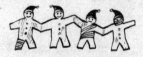

Thursday, 28 December 2006

I struggle with the concept of addiction – I think a lot of people do if they aren't addicts themselves. But it's hard to apply a rational thought process to people who can't be rational, whose minds have been taken hostage.

They're hospital staples. The patient being slowly suffocated to death by his smoking-induced emphysema, shivering in his wheelchair in the hospital car park while he alternates puffs from his cigarette and his oxygen tank. The alcoholic who's already lost his job and his family, warned by the doctors his liver is on the brink of cirrhotic no-return, but who still stops off at the pub for a post-discharge pint before he even makes it home.

And then there's Patient KM, a lady in her sixties, about to kill herself with sharon fruits. I've been asked to review her by the surgeons for an episode of post-menopausal bleeding. I read a clinic letter in the notes before reviewing her, then have to re-read it, assuming the consultant's secretary has been sniffing Tipp-Ex.

A decade or so ago KM underwent a gastrectomy* for stomach cancer and now has to keep to a strict diet, avoiding certain food types she can't digest. Top of the list is the persimmon, or sharon fruit – not exactly a Granny Smith, so an easy fruit to avoid. You might think.

Growing up in Malta, Patient KM's family tradition at Christmas has always involved eating sharon fruits, and this isn't a tradition she is prepared to let slide, despite her surgeon's threats.† She knew it wasn't an idle threat either; these little fuckers

---

* An –ectomy means a surgical removal. So removal of the stomach is a gastrectomy, male sterilization is a vasectomy, and private medicine is a cashectomy.

† God knows why – I've since tried one, and they're not much to write home about. Fibrous and flavourless, like a spherical raffia place mat. I don't think Terry's need to worry that Chocolate Orange sales are going to plummet in favour of sharon fruits any time soon.

have caused her to have five episodes of intestinal obstruction, ruining five separate Christmases – forming solid, concrete-like blockages in her colon and, on three separate occasions, requiring open surgery. The most recent was last week, when the surgeons sliced her open to squeeze the diospyrobezoar* out of her intestine, like a marble in a tube of toothpaste.

'It just wouldn't be Christmas without it,' she tells me, and I'm not sure whether she's talking about the fruit or her hospital admission for intestinal obstruction.

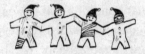

The next diary entry contains details of a medical procedure that may be extremely upsetting to read. If you wish to avoid this, please turn to page 68.

---

* Would you believe there's a medical term specifically and exclusively for a mass of undigested sharon fruit in an intestine? No wonder medical school takes so long, learning all this shit.

Friday, 29 December 2006

The concept of setting a Christmas 'out of office' doesn't really apply in medicine. Babies don't care about your plans to get acquainted with a large Baileys and the bottom of a tin of Celebrations – and medical emergencies don't get any less frequent just because Slade is belting out of every shop's PA system.

Prof Devereux's surgical termination of pregnancy list is definitely too time-sensitive to take a week off. I'm rota'd into theatre with Prof today, and first on the list is Patient SH, whose unbelievably sad story is the stuff of ethics textbooks – she's twenty-one and has a cardiac condition that means she's unlikely to live if she continues with her pregnancy. At fifteen weeks into her pregnancy her heart function has already significantly deteriorated and she's had to make the heartbreaking decision to end the pregnancy in order to save her own life.* So while the rest of the world was eating like a Tudor king, she was agonizing about the impossibly difficult decision

---

* Pregnancy puts huge demands on the body, and every organ has to adapt, from the liver to the lungs. The heart works around 50 per cent harder than before pregnancy, pumping much more blood around the body, and it's not something every single heart can cope with.

she'd made, and today, while everyone sleeps off their four-day hangovers in front of Bourne movie reruns, she's under general anaesthetic.

I've read her notes and know the story, but there's no discussion about it at all in theatre. Prof Devereux is chatting to the anaesthetist, arguing about who got treated the worst by the Christmas Rota Fairy. Instead of sitting on the stool to do the procedure, Prof turns to me and asks, 'Do you want to do it?'

I really, really don't. It feels so selfish to even think this – who am I to worry about *my* feelings, standing next to a patient going through the darkest, most traumatic day of her life? But the procedure is going to be grim beyond words – one more trauma for me to push down into a box that's already full to bursting.

D&Es are performed pretty rarely here; I've never even seen one before.* What will he think of me if I

---

* Most surgical terminations of pregnancy (TOP) are performed before twelve weeks' gestation, and are a much less complicated procedure, both technically and psychologically, using a small suction tube inserted into the neck of the womb. After thirteen weeks, surgical terminations of pregnancy would involve a D&E (dilatation and evacuation). This is a rare procedure, because terminations at such gestations are relatively uncommon, and the vast majority of them involve giving medication to induce a miscarriage. Some

say no? Turning down a training opportunity is not a good look. Should I tell the truth, that I'd find it too upsetting? It would be easier to tell him I'm drunk, or that I failed medical school and have been using a forged hospital pass for the last three years. What kind of doctor can't do their job because they're too soft?

It dawns on me that the inappropriately cheery pub banter with the anaesthetist is Prof's way of dealing with it. Doctors never debrief at home – if you don't even talk about it with the people in the same room, perhaps it helps you avoid thinking about it at all. Singing carols while London is blitzed around you.

Or maybe Prof just has a harder, tougher shell than me, a genetic stoicism, and this is something he can cope with day in day out, that simply doesn't pierce his armour.

If Patient SH is brave enough to go through this, then I should at least have the balls to step up for her. I say yes, even managing to sound keen. Prof clearly expects me to be grateful for the opportunity – it would be much quicker for him to do it himself rather than walk me through it. Besides, we're saving a life

---

patients, however, opt for the surgical route, under general anaesthetic, so as not to go through the added emotional distress of an induced second-trimester miscarriage.

here – without this procedure, the pregnancy will kill her – so who am I to think twice about doing that?

I wish I could say I was overreacting, that it was nowhere near as bad as I'd feared, but the truth is that every single step of it was absolutely horrible.

Dilating up the cervix with metal rods that feel almost barbaric in their size. Using an ultrasound to guide the instruments I put inside – a graphic, real-time reminder of what I'm doing. Grasping. Crushing. I see it all on the screen, but don't feel it in my hands – I feel it in my soul. Ripping. Pulling. There are things they never tell you when you apply to this specialty – they couldn't, you would run a mile. Praying it's over. It isn't. Pulling again. And again. Grateful for my surgical mask that hides my wobbling lip. Unable to reply to Prof Devereux's breezy matter-of-fact instructions with anything other than a robotic 'Mm-hm' in case my voice cracks. Repeating again and again in my head that we're saving a woman's life here. Suction. Scrape. Done. Minutes that felt like weeks.

I've read in the past that, when a patient chooses a late surgical TOP over a medical TOP, some of the burden of distress shifts from patient to doctor. Suddenly I understand. And then I feel guilty for making this in any way about me. It's nothing to do with me. I can go home, brood for a day or two, then allow it to fade into memory among the rest of the days I'd rather forget.

I'm jolted back into the here and now by Prof Devereux. 'Right, we're done! Wake her up!' he bouncily announces to the anaesthetist. The jollity is almost reassuring. 'Who's the next customer?'

'I need to head back to the ward, I'm afraid,' I say. But I don't. I need fresh air, or a quiet room. Even a noisy room – any room that isn't this one.

'No problem, you head off. I'll write up the notes.'

I stand up from the stool. He puts his hand on my shoulder and squeezes hard – he knew. This is our secret – I'm in the club now. He turns back to the anaesthetist and exhales.

'Are QPR playing today?'*

---

* I didn't put this diary entry in my first book because I couldn't face the thought of having to read it back again at the various proofing stages, and I felt very unsure about inflicting it on readers. I have since regretted this – it was one of the most impactful moments in my medical career.

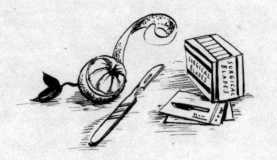

Fourth Christmas

Who's that you can see in his suit of magenta?
It's me – I've been soaked head to toe in placenta

Wednesday, 19 December 2007

Another missive from the powers-that-be, thunking into my pigeonhole with the friendly vernacular of a death threat.

Today's diktat – complete with crude Clip Art holly sprigs and so many semicolons per sentence it's practically a cry for help – informs all staff that the colour of scrubs will change this month from blue to red. Just like the cups in Starbucks! How fun! Maybe they'll also make us wear red velour hats with fluffy white trim instead of surgical caps, pointy-toed elfin winkle-pickers instead of theatre shoes, and replace the bleep's normal screech with the piano intro from 'All I Want for Christmas Is You'. I could totally get behind this.

But like a puppy in a gift box, this isn't just for Christmas – it's permanent. We'll be like those profoundly damaged breakfast-TV perennials who take Wizzard at their word and celebrate Christmas 365 days a year. Word soon spreads that the reason for the change isn't seasonal or sartorial – it's financial, naturally.*

---

* Scrubs aren't cheap – they need to cope with everything a hospital might fling at you, from all angles, often at great

I like my scrubs blue or green; they're a recognizable shorthand for 'medical professional' in a way that no other colour really is. At St Agatha's they insisted on different-coloured outfits for every profession – orange for anaesthetists, grey for midwives, purple for obstetricians and so on. When the whole team bundled in for an emergency alarm, it was like someone had called the Power Rangers.

Why are red scrubs the answer to our hospital's financial black hole? Is red a significantly cheaper dye? Are the department getting sponsorship from Virgin Atlantic? Nope. Blood doesn't show up on

---

speed. They're made of extremely high-quality cotton with a tightly knit high thread count, so the bugs can't get in (or out, knowing some of my former colleagues). But more expensive for the hospital than buying the scrubs is getting them cleaned, pressed and de-Ebola'd for the next person. On labour ward you get through a particularly large number: it's hard to emerge from any delivery unsplashed. You're basically front row for Shamu at SeaWorld, except Shamu has eaten a dodgy kebab and is suffering from chronic fin rot. And call them picky, but the average patient prefers it if, when a doctor knocks on their door, they don't look like they've just stepped out of a deleted scene from *Saw*.

red as easily, so they're hoping patients won't notice we're drenched in the stuff.*

[signature]

---

* Hospitals are always looking for ways to cut the cost of laundering so many scrubs. At one place where I worked they piloted a vending machine set-up, which saw each changing room fitted with a scrubs dispenser that, upon waggling your SCRUBZCARD™ (or whatever it was) over the electronic reader, would dole out a fresh set of top and trousers. It sounded great in principle, but unlike a regular vending machine, which hurls your Crunchie into the dispensing tray at such speed and force it gets reduced to sand, this chilled-out dude ejected its product glacially – not the speed a labour ward tends to function at. It was like waiting for the Bible to finish coming out of an inkjet printer.

Every member of staff was given a SCRUBZCARD™, and an allocation of three outfits a day from the machine. Nightshifts were fine – the card regenerated its credits at 12 a.m., so there were three sets available before midnight and three sets after, which was enough for all but the very sloppiest shift. Day shifts were more of a trial, getting by on just three pairs, so we started to game the system, learning to stockpile them. On clinic days when we didn't need to wear scrubs, we'd trot off to our robotic laundromat and relieve it of our full allocation, then hoard away our prized scrubs like those little glass pots from a chocolate dessert that might 'come in handy' one day.

Friday, 21 December 2007

On the one hand, my bleep has become a lot quieter since the new voice-activated switchboard system came in. On the other hand, it's virtually impossible for me to contact anyone else.

Presumably because the hospital is in a thunderingly posh area, the software company imagined the staff were on nodding terms with the landed gentry, and the system has been programmed to only recognize absurdly snooty accents. Every ward is full of doctors and nurses repeatedly honking a word into phone handsets in progressively posher voices. 'Theatre ... thurta ... thartaaaaah.' It's like an am-dram production of *Gosford Park*.

When you eventually manage to get switchboard's satanic robot to understand a word you've said, it's inevitably the wrong one. Today it would have been more efficient to get through to a radiologist with a couple of yoghurt pots and a length of string.

'Radiology.'

'Transferring you to Audiology. Or say: Cancel.'

'CANCEL!'

'Putting you through to Cancer Ward.'

Sunday, 23 December 2007

Like the gentle warm-down you do after a strenuous workout because it's bad for your body to go straight from sixty to zero, my gruelling nightshift is immediately followed by a day shift acting down a grade, as an SHO. I'm doing a good deed – the SHO who was meant to be on duty tonight recently lost her grandfather and has been refused compassionate leave, which is apparently restricted to first-degree relatives only. How nice to be informed that your nearest and dearest have some corresponding value attached to them, like a game of genealogical Top Trumps. And as if being denied compassionate leave wasn't enough, she couldn't even take the day off as annual leave, as she had given 'insufficient notice over the festive period'.

'As you know, this is standard policy' is HR's default line – as if being routinely malevolent is somehow better than dishing out acts of spite on an ad-hoc basis. On the bright side, this is relatively kind for them. They've been known to demand death certificates as proof in the past, and even state that only the loss of a partner, rather than their urgent admission to intensive care, were sufficient grounds to knock off work for a couple of days.

Despite management's unwavering insistence that she should miss her own grandad's funeral, we've managed to come through for this SHO and cobble together a little arrangement among ourselves. I'm staying on an extra six hours, and tonight's registrar is turning up six hours early. Ideally, she'd be able to grieve and support her family for more than a day, but it's better than nothing. How utterly depressing that the top floor have their own inflexible commandments, yet the rules and regulations that are supposed to protect rank-and-file staff are always gamed or ignored when the need arises.

But it's fine – relaxing almost! – working below my pay grade, even if it is for free. The registrar on the rota is a locum, naturally, and we both do our own thing for the most part. Out of courtesy, I let him know when I've admitted a patient, and we join forces twice to perform a couple of caesarean sections. I don't mention to him that I'm normally a registrar so as not to undermine him.

My half of the shift is over and we're about to say goodbye when he takes me aside and tells me I'm a good SHO.

'You should consider acting up as a registrar,' he says, shooting me the kind of patronizing grin I personally reserve for someone who tells me how clever their one-year-old is. 'Maybe in six months or so,' he adds.

Merry Christmas, you cunt.

Monday, 24 December 2007

Patient HL presents with an episode of post-coital bleeding. Inside, everything looks a bit . . . grazed. There's clearly a piece of her story missing – perhaps her boyfriend is that big yellow bloke from the *Fantastic Four* who's made entirely out of rock.

The actual answer is that, with no condoms available, she and her fella dipped into a Christmas selection box and improvised with a Mars bar wrapper – really embracing the 'play' aspect of 'work, rest and play'. The human desire to fuck seems to override any of our normal checks and balances. It's why you get people shagging in aeroplane toilets (a coffin that flushes!) or using a pepper mill in lieu of a dildo.

Luckily there's nothing to sew up for Patient HL

and it doesn't need packing.* I advise her to use less abrasive methods of contraception in future and, until it has totally healed, to take a break. By which I don't mean she should move on to KitKats.

(signature)

Tuesday, 25 December 2007

Fuck the halls with boughs of holly. It's four Christmases in a row and the depressing part is how normal it now feels. Routines are forming, like when a tree grows around a railing. The 7 a.m. bleary-eyed exchange of presents and a mince pie wolfed down while H pretends not to notice I've got one eye on the clock.

I didn't put up a fight when the Christmas rota came out this year. It's just the job, and someone has to do it. Maybe it appeals to the hero complex all

---

* As every boy scout knows, in the first instance you put pressure on a wound to stop it bleeding. This applies to vaginal lacerations too (although they tend to leave this part out of the boy scout handbook), and you apply this pressure by 'packing' the vagina with a length of gauze.

doctors pretend they don't have: Batman with a bleep. Plus there's that selfish buzz every member of our species is programmed to get after doing something good, like if you donate to a telethon or reunite a snivelling toddler with the teddy bear they've dropped. In the absence of a god tallying my actions on the heaven/hell ledger, it's something. But selflessness at hospital only serves to heighten my selfishness in other ways. Abandoning H, who has now stopped mentioning it because we have already had every possible permutation of the same discussion. Abandoning my family, who will never stop mentioning it. Even in death, they'll doubtless find a way via annual scheduled emails or a Ouija board.

Today's text from my mum says, 'Maybe we'll see you one year' – guilt, weaponized. I guess these days I'm just one of those people who doesn't celebrate Christmas, like a Jehovah's Witness, or a turkey.

On the drive into work, the biscuity-voiced radio presenter gives a shout-out to everyone working over Christmas, and I almost beep my horn in solidarity, before remembering I'm British. Then back to wondering if the car park will be free of charge today (obviously not).

I bustle in, look up at the labour ward board and sigh. 'Has anyone referred room eight to psych yet?'

Megan, one of the midwives, sighs back at me louder and tells me to take another look at the patient's info.

- 18 years
- Declined vaginal examination throughout labour as claimed to be '*virgo intacta*'
- For psych referral as claims child is 'son of god'
- Overseas patient: Nazareth
- Excessive number of visitors in room
- Baby male infant delivered at 00.00. Condition: stable

Ho ho *no*. It's only ten past eight and I'm already too tired for this shit.

Rather less 'humour' over on the gynae ward, where Patient HW has had a pretty grim week, the lowlights being emergency surgery for ovarian torsion* and a lingering post-op wound infection. I was desperate for her temperature to stay down so she could make it home at some point, to salvage a

---

* Please see footnote on page 44 of the paperback edition of *This is Going to Hurt*. OK, fine, just this once: ovarian torsion is when an ovary twists on its ligaments like a maypole, cutting off its blood supply.

bit of Christmas Day and stop December becoming a total write-off. I must have been an unexpectedly good boy this year because Santa has checked his list twice and given me what I asked for. Unfortunately, although Patient HW is now well enough clinically, there are logistical issues to deal with – she can't find anyone to drive her, and patient transport say there's no room on the back of their donkey.

Brook, one of the gynae nurses, goes full Chris Rea – minus the beard and the voice you'd get by accidentally gargling cement – and offers to drive her home. 'It's on my way anyway!' she says brightly, but another nurse quietly mentions that's not remotely the case. My icy heart thaws at this simple act of kindness.

I might sometimes go the extra mile at work, but – unlike Brook – I draw the line at going an extra seventeen on my way home. Brook tells the patient she'll be knocking off at 2 p.m. if she's OK to wait that long. 'Fine,' replies the patient. 'But I hope you're not expecting any money for the petrol.' That's the spirit.

Thursday, 27 December 2007

It's 4 a.m. and I crumple into a chair in the doctors' mess and make a noise like a deflating dinghy. Burton, one of the house officers, is curled up like a croissant on the sofa opposite me. 'How's your shift?' I ask.

He unfurls slightly and looks up at me – his body exhausted, his face puffy. He starts to speak but the effort is too much and he shakes his head and returns to his imaginary cocoon. Oh god. I was rather hoping to stare dead-eyed at the telly for half an hour, not counsel a traumatized colleague.

'Mate . . . are you OK?'

His head re-emerges, like the world's most lethargic meerkat.

'The vending machine's broken.'

Friday, 28 December 2007

'Insufficient sample' – the bane of a junior doctor's life. I get this weird dread when I look up a patient's blood result – like watching someone undress for the first time, or being in a McDonald's queue at 10.28 a.m. and praying you make it to the counter before the breakfast menu finishes.

It's always an urgent blood test – one that came from a patient with atom-thin veins, that took you fifteen attempts and left the patient looking like they'd just given a porcupine a hand-job. You cradle the precious test tube of blood like a white-gloved museum curator handling a first edition of the Old Testament, and with a quiet prayer you send it on its journey to the lab. And then it comes back as 'insufficient sample'. You can't shake the feeling that the lab technicians are gaslighting you – you *know* the hallowed ampoule was full to the brim. And even if it wasn't, murderers can be convicted on DNA evidence from a decades-old micro-fleck of spittle; can't the lab just live dangerously and have a bash at telling me a patient's clotting from 2.9 ml of blood rather than 3? But all you can do is bitch and moan at whoever's standing next to you, then go back to the patient for round two. A few more minutes' work for me, yet more track marks for the patient, but ultimately no real harm done.

It was much more irritating today when, reviewing a couple's results in infertility clinic, the semen analysis report showed 'insufficient sample'. Unlike a repeat blood test, there's nothing I can do for him here that wouldn't get me struck off. Instead the guy will have to book another appointment with the jizz deposit clinic, which – because there's no such thing as a semen emergency – will now be in the new year. Then, of course, he'll have to wait a month or so before seeing us back here in clinic – we can't discuss next steps until we have a complete set of results.

I'm about to break the news to them when my eyes drift a little further down the screen. Context! 'Scant sample, mixed with dirt, fluff, detritus. Please repeat.' Did he . . . wank into a hoover bag?

The patient seemed genuinely surprised he hadn't got away with it, but quietly admitted he had over-shot the container. No doubt with his grandmother's 'waste not want not' battle-cry ringing in his ears, he'd tried his best to scoop his issue back into the pot, bringing with it all the dust and DNA of whoever and whatever had gone before him.

'He does go a long way,' says his wife in a proud voice, like she was boasting about her child's grade three piano.*

---

* The long cumshot can be a useful diagnostic tool. (Is this the first time the word cumshot has appeared in a Christmas gift book?) A med school friend, now literally a brain surgeon,

I can't blame the guy for not having Olympic-archer accuracy – our lab doesn't have dedicated 'production rooms' as they're coyly described, so patients have to knock one out in the cubicles of the gents toilets. It can't be easy to bring yourself to the point of erotic ecstasy to the soundtrack of squeezing and straining from the cubicle next door. It's also fairly distracting for the hospital staff trying to get some 'me time' with their digestive system, knowing full well what the other cubicles moonlight as.*

---

managed to shoot himself in the eye one evening, and when what he initially thought was just minor irritation hadn't gone down a couple of weeks later, he popped to the doctor and was diagnosed with a strain of ocular chlamydia that hadn't given him symptoms in the usual postcode.

* A nurse who previously worked at an infertility clinic in the States told me they used to have a TV screen and DVD player. No word on the doubtless sub-motel-level pornographic delights available, but there was the chilling detail that the remote control was kept in a ziplock bag.

Back home, some units, including one I worked at, give you the requisite kit so you can collect the sample in the comfort of your own bedroom and bring in the specimen pot within an hour. Our instruction booklet said to 'keep the bottle at body temperature, for example in a trouser pocket, under your armpit or between your legs'. One man became the stuff of revolting legend and the headline act of many a doctor's dinner-party repertoire by interpreting this to mean 'inside your anus', which, in fairness, is undoubtedly body temperature.

As part of my BSc in Reproductive Medicine, I spent a couple of days working in a seminology lab, processing and testing the samples that came in. I meticulously followed the instructions the lab technician had given me: measuring the volume of the sample; transferring it to a new container; spinning it in the centrifuge to separate off the sperm from the unneeded fluid; chucking the fluid down the sink . . .

'What are you doing?!' yelped the lab tech. 'You've just thrown away the sperm!' I turned printer-paper white and scrabbled around the sink with my fingers.

She shrugged and toddled off to the computer to deliver the verdict: 'Insufficient sample'.*

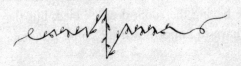

---

* As I was compiling this book, news came from China that could eradicate the 'insufficient sample' – although at perhaps a higher price to a patient's dignity. One hospital has announced the sperm-collecting machine, an object that looks a little like a customized water cooler with a hole for penile insertion. The machine will, using anatomically accurate vibrations and some frantic suction and thrusting, wank the patient off and collect anything they eject. The patient can then head back to work, complete with the psychological after-effects that come from having sex with a horny wastepaper basket.

Saturday, 29 December 2007

History hasn't recorded for us which Palaeolithic painter first mixed blue and yellow to make green, or blue and red to make purple. But it was Patient HC who discovered that if you bring a cinnamon and mulled wine plug-in air freshener into your delivery room for a bit of festive fragrance, rather than masking the unavoidable potpourri of blood, placenta, amniotic fluid and faeces, all forces somehow combine to create the most rancidly noxious stench imaginable. It hangs in the air like some kind of acrid death-gas in a James Bond film, its putrid cloud choking every airway, blunting every nerve ending. We're having the room deep cleaned, but they may well have to knock down the entire hospital.

Monday, 31 December 2007

My brother and I are both working in hospitals this New Year's Eve, so I call him for some sibling solidarity. We talk about our resolutions – I'm not

sure why I even bother, I don't think I've ever managed a lifestyle change that's seen out the Christmas
decorations. I don't blame myself, I blame January.
Everyone's wandering round like poorly reanimated
corpses and the weather would make Ernie Shackleton
think twice about popping down the shops for a pint
of milk; yet we choose this month for a bizarre act
of self-flagellation.

But once again, optimism triumphs over objectivity
and I've decided I'm going to have a pop at losing
a few pounds. How hard can it be? I barely have
time to eat anyway.

'Yeah, you probably should,' he replies. I was rather
hoping for a 'Don't be silly, you look great!' but with
a doctor's honesty added to a sibling's bluntness, this
was clearly unrealistic. He tells me he has some
important advice and my ears prick up. Perhaps he
went to some lecture at med school that I bunked
off? I'm already imagining myself svelter and am
looking forward to the little dopamine fist-bump any
time someone asks me if I've lost weight. ('Oh, I
dunno, maybe a bit?' I'll reply, while getting a
paper-cut off my own cheekbone.)

'Don't do what I did last year,' he says. 'You know
the "Taste the Difference" ready meals at Sainsbury's?'

I am aware of them, yes.

'Well, they're the fancy range, not the diet range. Took me until March to work out why I wasn't losing anything.'

Monday, 7 January 2008

Five weeks after meeting my accountant for my annual bollocking about record-keeping ('You'd do very badly in prison, Adam'), I'm still being diligent about holding on to receipts. This will all go to fuck at some point in February, but for now I'm a receipt-keeping poster boy for HMRC: the dry cleaning from when a patient accidentally pissed on my trousers in antenatal clinic; the £300 advanced life support course that is somehow mandatory for my job but for which the hospital provides neither the money nor the study leave (you can have that riddle for nothing, Rumpelstiltskin); a new stethoscope after my last one got slightly . . . blood-logged.

Labour ward isn't throwing too many dramas at me today, so I slope up to the on-call room for a bit of shut-eye. This is optimistic at the best of times, but today the bed – which has always erred on the Wormwood Scrubs side of luxurious – has been denuded of not just its bedding but also, mystifyingly, its mattress. I wonder where it's gone. Maybe it's being deloused? Maybe it blew away – it was certainly thin enough. Or maybe it's been sold to help with the hospital's deepening financial Mariana Trench. Given they replaced the canteen with a vending machine, nothing would surprise me now.

I'm not to be deterred – I'd probably accept the icy embrace of death if it was the only way I'd get a lie-down – so I have an exploratory rest on its wooden slats. I quickly realize this is incompatible with anything other than a chronic back injury, begrudgingly admit defeat and make my way back downstairs.

Before I leave, I stop off in what a London estate agent might describe as the en-suite, but which is quite clearly a broom cupboard that has been persuaded to masquerade as a toilet. As I'm sitting there, I notice the hand towel is gone too. Perhaps budget tightenings have also identified dry hands as a frivolous level of comfort – I fully expect to turn up one day and discover other luxuries have been removed, like light bulbs and walls.

I then realize, slightly too late, that there's no toilet roll either. Fuck. But invention is the daughter of necessity – I guess I'll just have to explain to my accountant why I've gone yet another year with no receipts.

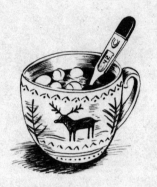

Fifth Christmas

I hang up my stocking, I lay down to sleep
Then shout 'fucking hell' at the sound of my bleep

Monday, 15 December 2008

I've spent the day in a distant hospital, examining students for their medical school finals, as a favour for an academic professor I've only met once. It's a non-optional favour, in the same way you'd be doing a speeding train a favour by jumping out of its path. Plus I've had to take the time from my precious supply of annual leave (something I don't mention to H). Still, I get to sit down all day and, for a nice change, nothing bad will happen if I take my eye off the ball. Well, maybe a dangerously negligent student qualifies as a doctor – no biggie.

My role in this low-budget gynaecology-themed version of *The Crystal Maze* is an assessment of the students' ability to perform a vaginal examination. Lying on the bed is a chunk of dismembered manne-quin, from belly button down to thigh stumps. It's like a magician's 'sawing the lady in half' trick gone hideously wrong, or Thing from *The Addams Family*'s randy aunt. I have a checklist of twenty actions the students have to perform, and I tick them off on my clipboard like a factory supervisor. My hapless charges are meant to treat the dummy like an actual patient, so among the fifteen ticks they need, they must introduce themselves, explain what they'd like to do, obtain consent, alcogel their hands and put on gloves.

I only failed one student, who missed out all the preliminary steps, instead marching into the room and wordlessly jamming his hand inside. Bareback.

Another student said to the dummy, 'Let me know if this is uncomfortable, sir,' and I very nearly burst out laughing. I put it down to his nervousness rather than ineptitude, as he immediately apologized about thirty times and asked me if he'd failed. He hadn't – there wasn't a box to tick for managing to identify the patient's gender.

Fifty or so students, a couple of litres of coffee, and a plate of custard creams later, I'm sitting in the pub with Kevin.

Kevin is a friend from university who texted me last week to say he'd handed in his notice and was leaving his job as a medical registrar at the end of the year to pursue his first love of acting. I responded as if the message said he was booked in to get an enormous spider's web tattooed across his face, and arranged to meet him in order to stage an intervention. 'It would be great to catch up before Christmas!' I replied – code for 'No! Don't go! Job before happiness, remember . . .'

He comes to meet me outside the hospital I'm

examining in; neither of us really knows the area. Lonely Planet are yet to release a set of guides to the shithole streets most NHS hospitals seem to find themselves on, so we duck into the first pub we see, a hundred yards from the revolving doors. This is our first mistake: it's the sort of pub the Krays might swerve because it looks 'a bit too stabby'. They've made the vaguest nod towards the festive season: half a canister of snow-spray applied to a couple of the windows that aren't boarded up, and some sun-faded Coronation-era paper chains rustling around the top of the bar.

Kevin has absolutely no interest in pep talks or discussing the merits and pitfalls of his momentous decision (stupid, but brave, I guess), so we focus on the more important business of getting drunk.*

'What white wines do you have?' I ask, trying to keep my voice as even as possible, so I'm not mistaken for a cop. The barmaid points one of her remaining fingers at a small row of individual plastic bottles of Chardonnay in the fridge and looks at me like I'm

---

* Unthinkable then, but just two years later I'd be out of the profession myself, and not even a naked, begging Chris Hemsworth could have persuaded me to change my mind.

Princess Margaret demanding a Brandy Alexander. I'm at the losing end of the beggar–chooser ratio here, so I thank her nervously, grab my Château Sarsons and Kevin's pint of lager, then ferry them over to the table Kevin has found. I sit down and the glasses make a disconcerting squelch as they settle into the sticky lake on the tabletop.

A few deep swigs of tepid battery acid later and I'm toasting his decision. I get halfway through asking for a mention in his first Oscars speech when a guy wanders over and puts a full pint of lager on our table. He explains that he's just got a round in, but his mate who's drinking beer has had to dash home. Would we like it? – he doesn't drink the stuff. We take a proper look at our mysterious benefactor – Daddy Warbucks he is not. He looks and smells like he's just been exhumed, and his fashion inspiration seems to come from Stig of the Dump's charity-shop toss-out pile: mismatched shoes, and a raincoat customized with enough stains to warrant its own CSI franchise. He sees we're mulling over how to answer, so chirps, 'Don't worry, it's clean!', which obviously adds considerably to our worry.

Kevin weighs up the odds, then gratefully accepts

his free pint, and our evening continues. I sit facing the room, and watch transfixed as, ten minutes later, our friend shambles over to another table, brandishing another pint of lager. I point it out to Kevin immediately. What is this guy's game? Given the toxic fumes radiating from his hell-coat, it would be understandable if his pals couldn't stand more than a minute of his company, but surely another friend can't have just left, unable to start their pint? Are we being filmed for an episode of *Secret Millionaire*?

Kevin moves his seat round so we can both keep an eye on what this guy is up to and, as a precautionary measure, puts his half-finished pint to one side. The man shuffles over to the bar and buys two pints of lager. He takes them back to his table and drinks a quarter of the first pint, followed by a quarter of the second. Next, he moves both glasses onto the floor, looks around, then bends down as if to tie his shoelace, before returning the first glass back to the table, filled to the brim.

This isn't the kind of pub in which you particularly want to be caught staring at someone, but we subtly reposition our seats to get a better view. In retrospect, ignorance was absolute bliss. It wasn't his shoe he was fiddling with, but his trouser leg which, when lifted up, revealed a catheter leg bag.* He was, horror of fucking horrors, opening the tap on the leg bag and allowing the contents to stream into the glass of beer, creating the world's most grotesque shandy.

I react more calmly than Kevin – unsurprising, given only moments before he'd been knocking back his free piss-beer like Paris Hilton on the Krug. I wonder out loud why the bloke might be doing this. And then whether any infectious diseases are potentially transmissible by drinking tramp urine. Some species of parasite perhaps? Kevin's response will sadly have to go unrecorded: he was far more concerned with racing to the toilet like Roadrunner on methamphetamine and forcing himself to purge. Not that his gag reflex needed much encouragement.

Guess I'll need to be more specific next time I tell H I'm going on the piss with Kevin.

---

* A discreet way to collect urine if you use a catheter is a thick plastic bag strapped to your leg. At the bottom of the bag is a valve (much like on a box of wine) to empty the contents into the toilet. Or a pint glass.

Wednesday, 17 December 2008

I've been unlucky enough to have drawn Mr Ribbons in the gynae Secret Santa. It's annoying to be forced to spend a tenner on someone who despises every aspect of my existence, from my handwriting to my knot-tying, and who I, as an entirely reasonable result, despise in return. I could get him something shit that he hates, but he'll only throw it away immediately and that's no victory at all.

H, presumably high on tinsel fumes, suggests I buy something thoughtful and nice, to try and build bridges. I explain that the only bridge I'd like to build has Ribbons' concrete-encased corpse in its foundations. I want to get something that will piss him off and inconvenience him so hard that it results in some kind of public breakdown.

'OK then. Buy him a guinea pig.'*

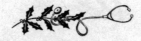

---

* I bought him a set of sandalwood styling wax and hair pomade. He is bald.

Monday, 22 December 2008

A couple of paediatric nurses are running around, recruiting volunteers to be Santa for an hour or two in the grotto they're running in outpatients. I'm shocked to even be asked – surely I'm far too young and slim to pass for Santa. I'd sooner work as a flambé chef on a Zeppelin, so I make my excuses. 'But . . . I'm Jewish!' If it's going to lumber me with extra Christmas shifts, it might as well get me out of this.

'The kids won't know!' the nurse replies, then pauses. 'Assuming you're not planning on showing them your penis?'

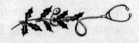

Tuesday, 23 December 2008

'And how frequently are you managing to have sex?' I ask the couple in infertility clinic.*

'About once a week,' the husband replies. 'It would be more but I work nights and I've been having a bit of trouble with the old downstairs neighbour.'

I always admire the talent for wordplay a patient will suddenly acquire when referring to their own body and its functions. This is definitely a new one. Not the bog-standard John Thomas, the nauseating <First name> Junior, or the ignominy of hearing a grown man saying 'front bottom'. Ever the professional, I don't flinch.

'Well, you needn't worry about your . . . neighbour,' I say, praying for a thesaurus to drop out of mid-air so we can all start speaking English again. 'Shift work can upset the body's natural rhythm and cause difficulties with sustaining erections.'

It turns out he meant his *actual* downstairs neighbour, who's been having noisy building work done during the day, so they're staying with his parents

---

* Not an unreasonable question – some people seem to think a monthly fumble will cut it. (The answer is ideally every day or two during the woman's fertile window.)

and sleeping on the sofa, limiting their romantic opportunities.

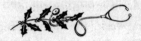

Thursday, 25 December 2008

Christmas number five – I think we're getting into Norris McWhirter territory here. H is with family: plans made before my rota was even announced.

Mr O'Hare is on call for labour ward so, as tradition holds, he appears at lunchtime to cut the turkey in his casual wear. To him it may well be 'this old thing', but to me it's the kind of get-up I'd wear to accept a knighthood. He does it with great ceremony in the staff room and insists the scrub nurse stands opposite him and passes each utensil as he needs it ('Fork please, sister'). It's funny and rather sweet, bringing a much-needed home-from-home atmosphere.

'See,' I say to Karen, an SHO doing her first Christmas Day on call, 'it's fun here at Christmas – we're like a work family!' She's unconvinced, preferring the idea of her *family* family, and asks me if there's a blood test for Stockholm syndrome.

The turkey ritual manages to briefly circumvent the usually immovable barrier between consultants and the rest of us. Well, to a certain extent; we're not going to start texting each other jokes and braiding one another's hair. This is the season of goodwill, yes, but there are boundaries: we still call him 'Mr O'Hare' – calling him Gerry would be like calling the Queen 'Liz'.

After a few minutes of turkey and semi-forced chatter, he pulls me aside to run through the labour ward board. There's a patient at 7 cm dilation going for a vaginal breech delivery.*

'You confident with those?' he asks, and I reflexively blurt out that I am, so he nods and strides off home. I'm not remotely confident. I've only delivered one vaginal breech before, and that was an uncomplicated birth that didn't require forceps. If I'm bleeped to do a breech forceps delivery, I'll be doing it for the first time and unsupervised.

---

* The majority of breech (bottom-first) babies are born by caesarean section, which is generally thought to be the safest method of delivery for the baby. In a patient with no other risk factors and a unit with suitably experienced midwifery and obstetric staff, vaginal breech should always be offered as an option. In a minority of vaginal breech births, the body will deliver but the head gets stuck, at which point forceps are needed to deliver the head fairly smartish.

My mind goes straight to the worst-case scenario, then plays it all forwards: the family for whom Christmas becomes the day on the calendar they dread forevermore – every carol they hear, every cutesy festive film and stodgy mince pie a reminder of the time a registrar blagged it rather than admitted he wasn't experienced enough.

Maybe if it wasn't today I'd have answered Mr O'Hare differently. I'm not even allowed to use his first name – it's going to go down like a semen soufflé if I'm the one who takes him away from his family at Christmas. And that's exactly what will stick in his mind when I'm applying for consultant jobs and someone taps him up for a reference. 'Kay – I remember the chap. Couldn't deliver breeches.' Not the thousand days I stayed late, or the thousand emergencies I handled on my own, but the one time I admitted I was out of my depth and asked for help.

I hide in the toilet, looking up on my phone how to deliver an aftercoming head with forceps – not the first time I've been in a cubicle with a phone in one hand looking for videos, but the first time quite like this. Unsurprisingly there is no such thing on YouTube, but I do find a useful PowerPoint presentation – it was designed to compare techniques, but comes in handy as the medical equivalent of a York Notes crammer.

I feel a bit more prepared . . . but not enough. I spend an hour seeing patients in triage, feeling like I'm about to vomit up everything I've eaten in the last five years. The midwife supervisor gives me fair warning: the breech patient will start pushing in half an hour. It's all getting slightly too real now. After a few agonizing minutes weighing up the relative horror of each scenario, I bottle it and call Mr O'Hare. As his mobile rings, I'm extremely aware that if I'd just told him in the first place, he'd have been far less irritated than he will be now that I've let him get all the way home, his fork doubtless poised over its first pig-in-blanket.

I'm halfway through my stuttering apology when Mr O'Hare hushes me to say he's just downstairs in his office. Did I really think he was going to go home with an undelivered breech on labour ward? I don't know whether to feel relieved or insulted, but relieved edges it.

The mum starts pushing and I'm sitting at the nursing station with Mr O'Hare, waiting for either the midwife to call us in to help or for a baby's cry. Happily it's the latter – though it does mean I needn't have fucking called him in the first place. I apologize for wasting his time but he says he'd much rather be called a thousand times for something that was fine in the end than not be phoned once about something that went wrong.

'I've done the job thirty years and it still scares me sometimes,' he confides, and it's the first time I've ever heard a consultant say something like that. I feel reassured hearing it from the safest pair of hands on labour ward. Maybe we're not so different after all (Aston Martin aside). I respect him for showing his vulnerability and I like to think it's been a significant moment for us both.

He stands up to leave.

'Merry Christmas, Adam.'

I pause.

'Merry Christmas, Gerry.'

He looks at me like I've just announced I have sex with household pets, and walks off. Bollocks.

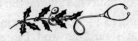

Sunday, 28 December 2008

Normal rules don't seem to apply in hospital. The clothes are different, the food is different, the language is different and, gallingly for Brits, queuing is out. Watching someone else get wheeled off while you've been waiting longer must be frustrating, but that's just how it goes.

I feel sorry for the patient doing the whole 'I was here first' routine to Linnie, a Welsh terrier of a midwife supervisor who takes absolutely zero shit from anyone.

'Oh, I'm so sorry, madam,' Linnie replies. 'But I think you're confusing my labour ward with a deli counter.'

Wednesday, 31 December 2008

Last nightshift of the run. I phone the SHO to check he's not drowning in a sea of patients in A&E. There's only one left, so I offer to review her and clear the department. 'It's just a six-weeker with bleeding,' he tells me.

As soon as I've hung up I'm annoyed with myself for not pulling him up on that – no one's *just* anything. It's no less of a pregnancy for this patient than for anyone else, however many weeks advanced.

I'm about to call him back when a patient taps me on the arm.

'That applies to *you* too.' Excuse me?! She points to a 'No Mobile Phones' notice on the wall, its laminate edges looking as tired and frayed as I do, informing us that phones interfere with sensitive medical equipment. From the abject disgust on her face, you'd think I had a tourniquet round my arm and a syringe full of heroin dangling out. (Though I'm not ruling that out by the end of the shift.)

I want to tell her the truth, that mobile phones interfere with fuck all, and we only have the signs up so patients aren't sitting around crowing into them all day, driving the rest of us mad with their inane conversations. But that would rather give the game away, and would also mean this conversation lasting much longer than my nerves can stand, so instead I paint on my best meek face, mutter an inaudible apology and head down to A&E.

Patient EN definitely isn't 'just' a six-weeker. I can tell from their raddled faces and raw eyes that she and her husband have been crying. They've only stopped because they've run out of tears and energy. They're in their early thirties, this is their fourth cycle of IVF and the one that's got the furthest. I want to say they're lucky to be in an area that offers three rounds of IVF on the NHS – edge a few miles south, and it's one try then bye – but if three have failed then all it means is three times the agony. They've ploughed every penny they'd saved for a deposit on a house into this fourth cycle. All their chips on the same square, both financial and emotional, and here I come, the croupier who's going to sweep them away.

I scan her and tell them the uterus is empty, that the bleeding very sadly does mean the end of the pregnancy.

Their desperation is heartbreaking. 'But we had a normal scan a week ago. Can you have another look? Maybe you missed it?' I know I haven't missed anything but the patient is right there, begging for a final ray of hope. Her eyes searching mine, the husband stock-still next to her, frightened to speak in case it makes the unthinkable true. I repeat the scan, have a second look, pass her some paper towel to clean off the ultrasound gel, and shake my head.

Amid the grief, she searches for answers and explanations. She asks if there's any way the scan she had last week could have caused this? I know she wants me to say yes – she needs there to have been a reason, something they could do differently if there were to be a next time. I've got nothing for her.

I talk about next steps. It's a speech I've given so

many times that I fail to stop myself before saying, 'There's no reason you can't try again.' But there is, isn't there? Unless they win the lottery. We live in a world of lotteries, of being in the right place at the right time, of all kinds of sheer luck – and theirs has probably just run out.

There's a sudden racket from the other side of the blue curtain – crowd noises, general chaos – someone's put the volume up on the TV. I realize before my patient what's about to happen and steel myself in an emotional brace position. *Five!* screams the TV. *Four!* Everyone in A&E joins in. Louder now. *Three! Two! One!* Cheering, whooping, party poppers, stamping feet, Auld Lang Syne.

'I'm sorry,' I say. About the noise, about their baby, about the IVF, about other people being happy. 'I'm so sorry.'

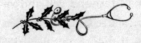

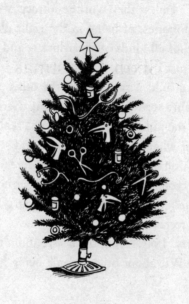

Sixth Christmas

Security break up their fifty-eighth fight
Happy Christmas to all, and to all a good night

Tuesday, 15 December 2009

'Was Daddy there when I was born, Mummy?'

'No, he wasn't, baby-who-Adam-has-just-delivered. You see, Mummy went into labour while Daddy was out at a Christmas party.'

'So he didn't make it to hospital in time?'

'Well, darling, he made it to hospital in time, but he was so drunk that he whipped out his cock when the doctor was putting the forceps on your head, and they had to call security to boot him out.'

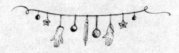

Wednesday, 16 December 2009

H was genuinely surprised I made it to the theatre in good time for the start of *A Christmas Carol*, probably because overrunning shifts have meant I've missed the first half of almost every other play we've seen this year. Unfortunately, when we took our seats in the stalls I immediately fell asleep. After eight labour ward shifts on the trot, my brain had clearly declared it an emergency and just powered down.

H prodded me awake the first couple of times I nodded off, before the gentleman to my left took over. I may not be the silent sleeper I'd assumed I was. Sensing the murderous intentions of other paying customers in our immediate radius, we headed home at the interval so as not to cause any more disruption. Still, makes a nice change to miss the second half of a play for once.

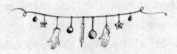

Saturday, 19 December 2009

This job is really adding to the 'other skills' section of my CV – today, *magistrate* joins the list alongside *social worker* and *cleaner*. I meet midwife Georgette and Prof Pruitt (a nice Australian consultant who works on labour ward with the approximate frequency of Halley's Comet) in closed session to discuss the case of Patient DH.

The defendant has been on the antenatal ward for

the last three weeks with major placenta praevia*
and constant vaginal spotting. Fingers crossed she
won't do anything too dramatic for the next five
weeks, at which point baby will be near enough fully
cooked, and we can perform a caesarean under
controlled circumstances. There are four units of
crossmatched blood for her on labour ward at all
times, in case things kick off and we need to deliver
her in a hurry. She's effectively sitting in a prison
cell with an unexploded mine in the corner.

The complainant, Patient TW, has informed me on
my ward round that the defendant is running a
'Christmas card racket' from her bed, drawing
'shoddy cards' and selling them to other hospital
residents in aid of 'some unnamed charity'. 'It's not
what the NHS is about, is it?' she asks.

My 'And . . . ?!' goes down like a turd in her tea,
so in the absence of a formal ombudsman system,

---

* Placenta praevia means the placenta is lying too low and
getting in the way. Major is the most severe type, where it
sits right over the neck of the womb, and baby has to be
delivered via the emergency exit. Because of the risk of heavy
bleeding, patients who have recurrent symptoms are often
kept on the ward for their own safety, hopefully having a
boringly uneventful time, until baby's far enough along to be
delivered.

or – as I suspect the patient would prefer – my immediate dismissal for insubordination, I promise to speak to my consultant.

It's fair to say that, no, the cards are not of the highest quality, like something a kid might bring home from school that you'd discreetly bung into the recycling rather than display on the Smeg door.

Our supergrass is wrong about the charity being unnamed, however: it is mentioned on the back of the cards, and the defendant has collected all the money she's raised (£30) in an envelope to pay in once she's out of hospital. Whether she actually does that or not, we cannot guarantee, but as frauds go, I doubt it would give Rumpole too much of a migraine.

Our verdict is unanimous: the defendant should be acquitted of all charges. She's locked up in hospital over Christmas and when she's not bored out of her mind, she's probably worrying about the ticking time bomb nestled in her uterus, and is doing a nice thing to keep herself busy.

Talk turns to other enterprising inpatients. Prof tells us when he was a junior doctor they found out one of the antenatal patients had been doling out blow jobs in her cubicle to male inpatients – apparently at fairly competitive rates.

'What did you do?!' Georgette and I ask in unison.

'I think we just gave her a side room.' Registering our mouths hanging open like the back of a bin lorry, he adds, 'This was back in Australia, of course,' as if that somehow explained it.

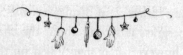

Sunday, 20 December 2009

Out for annual Christmas drinks with school friends. Well, annual for them. The fact I'm not on a shift is met not so much with surprise, but like we're in a horror film and I died in a fire five years earlier.*

---

* At the degree ceremony they never mention the huge impact medicine will have on your social life. It's not simply missing things because of your rota. It's more that if it's 5 p.m. and someone starts bleeding out on labour ward, then you stay and sort it out. There's no one who can take over from you, so you end up leaving a few hours late – this means you're routinely texting people to cancel on drinks or dinner at the last minute. By the third time you've cancelled on the same person, you've become the 'flaky friend' and you stop getting invited out. Your social circle contracts before your very eyes, like a miserable magic trick.

Everyone seems disproportionately happy to see me. I don't owe them any money so maybe they're finally warming to my revolting anecdotes after all these years?

Oh no, it's not that. Now we've hit our late twenties they only care about my professional qualifications – everyone's starting to procreate and to them I'm a one-man antenatal clinic. They all but form a queue to ask me questions. 'Is it true walking under power cables can make the umbilical cord get trapped around baby's neck?'* 'Is there a vegan alternative to breastfeeding?'†

Jack asks me what I think about 5D scans – he and his wife are 'thinking of getting one done privately' and wonder if they're worth the money. Typically, if you have to ask whether something medical is 'worth the money', the answer is no – unless it's a pioneering operation to reattach a severed head. But nobody wants to hear me smart-mouth my way out of awkward questions. Instead I say I

---

* What the fuck?
† Also, what the fuck? Surely breastfeeding is the single most natural thing in the world? And – chapped nipples aside – no animals are getting harmed. Plus, this baby's sole source of nutrition in utero was blood, which isn't an especially vegan start.

don't really know enough about them to answer, but wonder aloud how the private sector are able to offer two entire additional dimensions.

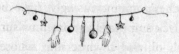

Monday, 21 December 2009

Giving my bleep the same hopeful look I give the front door when I'm waiting in for a parcel and need to leave the house. Silence. Today of all days, nothing. Surely labour ward can serve me up one of its usual time-consuming 8 p.m. emergencies to give me an excuse to miss the dreaded Christmas Ball.

'Ball' is stretching the word to the very perimeter of its meaning – the Met Gala it is not. This annual St Dominic's tradition is held in the greasy, windowless basement function room of a local two-star hotel. H has declined to be my escort on the grounds of 'absolutely no way', so I will be going alone or, if the stars align (assuming they aren't too busy pointing the three kings to Bethlehem), detained at work.

But alas, my prayers go unanswered – you'd have

thought god might have embraced the novelty of someone desperate for a medical crisis, given most people are begging for the opposite. I plod to the locker room and change into my cobbled-together 'smart clothes'; an increasingly tight but not yet indecent black suit that has somehow survived since medical school, and a white shirt whose stains are invisible if I don't take off my jacket. Plus the *pièce de disgustance*, my trusty Christmas tie. Its edges are tatterdemalion and poor Rudolph looks like he could do with a few weeks at Champneys. I give the button an exploratory press, assuming its battery is long-perished. But while my TV remote needs fresh batteries every other week, this fucker seems to have seen out half a decade. It's definitely entering death-rattle phase – the noise it makes isn't instantly recognizable as 'Jingle Bells' but more of a low, slow, droning honk, like a tuba being buried at sea. I reach for a stitch-cutter blade and euthanize the bastard thing out of its misery. No such reprieve for me: my obligatory entertainment awaits.

The ball is of course – by all objective measures – terrible. We are greeted – and I use this term loosely because, despite their elf hats, the waiting staff have facial expressions normally reserved for root canal surgery – with a plastic flute of warm sub-cava.

For dinner I receive a starter of what was presumably mozzarella in a previous life, surrounded with limp, geriatric supermarket salad leaves, like liver failure on a plate. Because I'd failed to pre-order the vegetarian main course, I get an 'I'll see what I can do' from the nearest elf, delivered as convincingly as a 'you look great' from an ex. What eventually arrives is my starter, again. Then there's a dessert of chocolate slurry so faeculent that I scan the room looking for the dog responsible.

During coffee-coloured liquid, we are treated to a thirty-minute speech from the medical director, which is only marginally less interesting than the teaching session he gave last month on polypharmacy in the elderly. Finally there's a ceilidh band. (Why? If we were much further away from Scotland, we'd be in the sea.)

Despite my initial Scroogings, it's actually an enjoyable evening, entirely out of step with the sum of its parts. I get to talk to my doctor, nurse and midwife colleagues – and not just to impart medical information. They're all so different tonight, and it's not only the tuxes and evening dresses. They're duplicates of their normal selves – only more animated, more fun, more human. Once we put our scrubs on, it's clearly all role-play. I realize I hadn't really thought of them as people before – with lives and interests and a sense of humour – and feel bad for assuming I was the only one with a personality (such as it is). Especially as that's precisely what frustrates me about the other players in this game – the patients and the politicians, forgetting that we're human.

'We should hang out more often,' I say to one of the gynae nurses and we clink glasses. I really mean it, but we both know the truth: we won't have the time. Work will make sure of it.

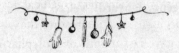

Wednesday, 23 December 2009

At this time of year the hospital is always Locum Central. With so many new faces on labour ward, it's a bit of a game of Russian roulette, with the barrel of the gun pressed against the clammy temples of the patients' heads. Will they have overstated their experience by five years in the hope of blagging it and getting maximum Christmas spending money, while I end up doing two people's jobs to keep a floor full of mothers and babies alive? Or will I get a ludicrously experienced gynae consultant,* and spend my shift drinking tea and reading trashy magazines in the coffee room, the ones with headlines like 'Slay Ride: Santa murdered my husband!' and 'My daughter's a minotaur!'

Heather, the SHO about to depart for the evening and hand over to a locum, nudges me as she spies a figure walking down the corridor. 'That's a bad sign.'

'What is?' I ask.

She points at the guy loping towards us, wearing a locum agency lanyard. 'Velcro shoes . . . can't tie knots.'

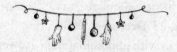

---

* This is actually not as unusual as you might think, thanks to the UK system's treatment of foreign-trained doctors and the endless hoops they have to jump through to get a substantive job here. It's at best zealous and at worst xenophobic.

Friday, 25 December 2009

There are busy shifts, there are very busy shifts, and then there are apocalyptic, balls-to-the-wall shifts where you'd gladly swap places with the turkey crisping away at gas mark 4.

It's not until we're nearing the end and I meet Patient GA in her Christmas jumper that I even remember what day it is, like when you get out of the cinema and it's still light, or come round from a thirty-year coma.

'Where do you work?' I ask, seeing from her notes she's a paediatric nurse. She tells me and it turns out I'd done an attachment there as a medical student, so we swap stories about the mad 'Paternoster' lift system.[*]

She's come in with abdominal pain at twenty-eight

---

[*] This is a bizarre, antiquated, open-fronted lift that moves constantly between floors on a wire like a ski lift, or a toaster in a hotel breakfast buffet. When it gets to your floor, if you don't leap off in time, you're doomed to stay on it, eventually finding yourself travelling through an eerie, pitch-dark, terrifying roof space that seems to exist outside of linear time, before the lift continues its journey and goes back down again. When up in the void, you generally feel the need to mutter a quick prayer that you'll make it back safely: 'Our father . . .' – or *pater noster* in Latin.

weeks, and is accompanied by her mother. I examine her and strap her onto the CTG machine, while mum goes outside to do what I probably should have done four hours ago – phone home and check in on everyone's Christmas Day. Once the prospective grandmother is out of sight, Patient GA leans in and whispers conspiratorially, as if she's about to tell me she isn't actually pregnant.

'I've not worked there since July,' she says. I raise an eyebrow. 'It just got too busy, too stressful, too horrible. I haven't worked as a nurse at all since then, but I can't face telling my parents.' I can totally understand – a combination of shame, a feeling of failure, a dereliction of duty; letting down the people who invested so much in your career.

'It's not *why* I got pregnant, but it gives me a while to work out what I'm going to do next . . .' She cocks an ear as she hears familiar footsteps trooping over. 'I'm just going to tell them I decided not to go back after maternity leave.'

Her mum bounds back into the cubicle with news of who won Monopoly and the terrible traffic Brian ran into on the M4 – we clam up as though teacher has just walked in. The pain has settled and her CTG is normal, so I send her home.

I drive back home myself, five hours later and two

hours late, covered in fluids that would give the most specialist fetish clubs in Berlin a run for their money, and wishing I had some suture material to secure my eyelids open. But I've still got a smile on my face – I delivered six healthy babies today to six healthy mothers. The job still gives a lot back, despite all it takes from you: the Christmases, the social life, the family life. I wonder what I'd tell *my* parents if I ever left. Probably nothing – how else could I hang on to my cast-iron excuse for skipping Christmas at their house? Join the army?*

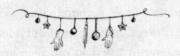

---

* When I left medicine, I *did* tell my parents – not immediately, but within a couple of weeks. In fairness, I don't generally speak to them much more often than that (I'm not a Kardashian). But I didn't tell them *why* I'd left – that I couldn't hack the job. I gave the impression I was doing really well after the break-up of my relationship and using this change of circumstances as a catalyst to finally follow my dream of becoming a writer. They reacted as if I'd just announced I was moving to Alpha Centauri to knit scarves out of space dust.

They only found out my real reasons seven years later, when my first book came out.

Wednesday, 30 December 2009

'And what's *your* name?' I ask the ten-year-old accompanying his mum to antenatal clinic.

'Coyle,' he says.

'That's a nice name,' I reply, my child-communicating skills still second-to-none. I'll be asking who his favourite member of ABBA is next, or whether he got a spinning top for Christmas.

'It's because I got pregnant with him when I had a coil in,' his mum informs the room, loud enough to induce labour in a Serengeti elephant.

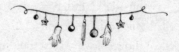

Thursday, 31 December 2009

I'm not a huge fan of forced fun and, at those rare parties my rota allows me to attend, I'll always look for an excuse to leave early. Not much really cuts it when it comes to escaping before midnight on New Year's Eve, but Patient CW has just about aced it with the fairly rock-solid excuse of going into labour. She's got twins on the way and is booked in for a caesarean next week, but it seems her babies are anxious to put in an appearance before the last glass of champagne has gone flat.

She's huffing and puffing away, but she's only a couple of centimetres dilated, so I explain there's no great hurry – we'll do the caesarean at some point tonight.

'So it could be *any* time tonight?' asks her husband.

I say it depends on what else might be happening on labour ward and making sure it's safe and convenient for the paediatrics team and anaesthetist – but at time of press, labour ward isn't madly busy. He looks at me furtively, as if he's about to offer to sell me some weed outside Camden Town tube station, and asks if the babies might be delivered at midnight. It's a couple of hours away so I tell him it's not unfeasible. He gets that conspiratorial look about him again – is he planning to eat these children?

'So . . . technically,' he says, 'you could deliver one just before midnight and the other just after, so they'd be born in different years?'

He looks at his wife for her take, and she agrees it's the best idea ever. This is because it *is* the best idea ever. How can I not be in on it? Rewarding as the job may be, I'm not immune to the thrilling prospect of featuring in a local paper as the obstetrician who transcended the accepted workings of time. This is as close to fame as I'm likely to get: I'm never going to appear on *Big Brother* – if I wanted to share a sweaty dorm with people whose mental age was twelve I'd have become a scoutmaster.

Also, why not? Both babies' CTGs are totally normal and she's not contracting away too dramatically, so I can't see any negative implications for the patient, the babies or my GMC registration – only the best anecdote in the history of the world, and a set of twins who spend the rest of their lives explaining why they were born in different years.

I liaise with the anaesthetist and theatre staff about getting mum round to theatre for half eleven – enough time for her spinal block, and then I can deliver the babies right on cue. There's enough of a buffer zone in the timings; I can rush a baby out in under a minute for a crash section, or equally well take the fifteen-minute scenic route, cauterizing every tiny blood vessel so I barely spill a drop.

Game on. I am already privately composing my quote for the press and deciding which way I should stand for the photographer. Do I even have a best side? Should I ask them to airbrush my dark circles or leave them in for that 'tired yet valiant doctor' authenticity?

I'd forgotten, however, that nothing ever goes to plan on labour ward. They should translate that into Latin, make it the motto of the Royal College of Obstetricians and Gynaecologists and chisel it above every delivery suite doorway. You can't guarantee there'll be time for a shit or a sandwich during your shift, so I don't know why I thought this stood a chance of working out. Cue a post-partum haemorrhage on the postnatal ward, a ventouse in room four and a patient's boyfriend in room nine having an episode of micturition syncope.* It was half one by the time I delivered the little bastards.

Maybe next year – I certainly don't need a clairvoyant to tell me I'll be working.†

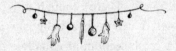

---

* Fainting while having a piss is surprisingly common in men, and usually nothing to worry about. Lots of guys wake up on a bathroom floor with an Armitage-Shanks-shaped dent in their forehead, wondering why their knob's hanging out but they still have their wallet and car keys. See also coital cephalgia: a terrible headache at the point of orgasm that makes patients think they've had an aneurysm.
† But I wasn't. The year that followed showed me what my limits were, and tested me far beyond them. By the next Christmas I was already on my way out of the profession.

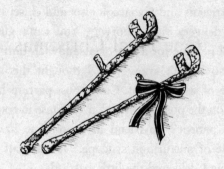

One Final Christmas

There's always something *not quite right* about other people's Christmases. My partner J and I alternate families – one year on, one year off – moaning about how wrong everything is.

J's family start the day with a Buck's Fizz at breakfast, which is plainly deranged. We're not at an airport. The rest of the breakfast is, for some unintelligible reason, made up of a variety pack of cereals, so he and his (grown adult, I should add) siblings can fight over the same two little boxes. Presents are disseminated – a stocking containing a hundred tiny bits of tat rather than a nice, *quick*, single gift. Each item in the stocking, even if it's a vodka miniature, is intricately wrapped and adorned with a fucking bow, except for some reason the tangerine and the apple. An apple? The first time I saw one being produced from the toe of a stocking, I assumed it was for the horse that was about to trot in, because by that point nothing would have surprised me.

They sit in a circle like they are about to summon

Jesus himself to cook the sprouts, then – in reverse-age order – open one present at a time, a process that takes three hours even with a strong tailwind. Lunch is served at what should be dinnertime and involves *starters*. Who needs starters? Hurry up and get me my potatoes. And what the fuck is bread sauce? And why does it look like watered-down loft insulation? Dessert has to wait – even though it's basically Boxing Day by now – because first it's the sixteen-round quiz that I have spent every evening for the last fortnight watching J painstakingly assemble.

Luckily, this year we are spending Christmas at my family's house so everything is entirely nice, normal and proper. J somehow can't get his head round this and is constantly complaining that no one's performing a trombone solo while the turkey is carved, or whatever bullshit his family do.

I realize Christmas is partly about creating your own traditions, so I've squeezed a new one into our family. Every year we bring our nieces and nephews presents they adore (to ensure we're always their favourite uncles) and their parents hate (because ahahaha). We've done the toys that reach jet-engine decibels, toys so messy they've resulted in the repainting of walls and incineration of rugs, and toys that take a thousand parent-hours of construction

– but this year we've really excelled ourselves. Each of the four Junior Kays gets an eight-foot-tall, wonderfully cuddly teddy bear, a good ten times the volume of an average six-year-old. The kids are naturally in love at first sight, while my brothers struggle to calculate how these gigantic velour mutants will fit in their houses, let alone their cars, and begin plotting my urgent death.

My sister Sophie spent last night working on labour ward* and emerges from bed just in time for 'celebration ice cream' – the perfectly normal concoction my mother makes every year with candied fruit and rum. I conduct a full-blown autopsy of everything that happened on her shift: the caesareans, the ventouses, the patient who burst her stitches on the postnatal ward, the news from A&E about the woman who collapsed at midnight mass (she said she'd been praying too hard; toxicology said she'd been drinking out of her hip flask even harder). My brother has to dash off to his out-of-hours GP session, so I go upstairs for my entirely normal afternoon nap slightly earlier than usual, to ensure I have enough energy for the traditional – and again,

---

* She works in obs and gynae, which makes me suspect she didn't read my last book.

absolutely normal – midnight viewing of *Silence of the Lambs*.

J follows me upstairs and crouches next to me as I plomp down onto the bed. He doesn't say anything, just stares at me for a while, his eyes gleaming, the beginnings of a smile.

'What?' I say. 'It's perfectly fine to go to bed halfway through Christmas Day.'

'No, not that – although no, it isn't,' says J. 'You miss it, don't you?'

I prop myself up in bed and look at him.

'I saw your face when you were talking to Sophie,' he continues. 'You miss working in hospital over Christmas!'

I laugh a little too hard, before saying, 'Of course not!'

But we both know I do. I really, really do.

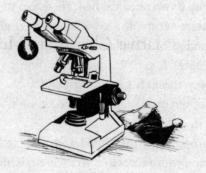

Alternative Christmas Message

I think there's room for a new tradition at this time of year. Or we could just elbow out an old one. Watching Her Maj peer into the autocue for ten minutes of plummy platitudes, maybe. The globally resented Boxing Day walk, accompanied by relatives who are trying to be jolly despite the vengeful, constant throat-punch of a near-fatal hangover. Or Christmas pudding – that claggy nightmare where the six-pence is the most edible part. Slosh on some extra brandy and let's burn that sultana dungheap down for good.

My proposal would be to find some way of acknowledging the fact that at Christmas, half a million NHS staff will be spending the day at work – from porters to physios to pharmacists – and the majority who aren't will soon be sacrificing their Boxing Days and New Year's Eves. Working on the front line, invisible to most of us, while we calculate whether we can physically manage to consume any more brie. (Yes, just eat it with a grape and it's practically a health food.)

Maybe as we sit around in our party hats, about to risk our lives on a half-defrosted King Prawn Ring, we can bow our heads in prayer. Not to thank the god who, let's be honest, has probably done more harm than good every single week since that very busy first one. But instead to thank the people without whom we might not all be here; the people who will finally get home at midnight and pick at leftovers from the fridge while you've long surrendered your senses to a carbohydrate coma.

Better still, let them know you're grateful. It's easier than you'd think to make an NHS employee's day, especially at Christmas. Send a card to your GP, to the outpatient clinic you visited, or the ward you were on. They *will* remember you (it might take a moment because they meet a lot of people) and your message might just turn a bad day into a reminder of why they do their job.

If you've been lucky enough to enjoy optimum health and haven't needed the services of the NHS, remember that your invincibility is on a timer and your good fortune can be shared in other ways. Make a donation to your local neonatal unit or a hospice or medical charity*. Give blood. Join the Organ Donation Register.

If you don't have the energy or the means to help in those ways, there is still something you can do for the beleaguered staff missing Christmas Day at home. Stop sticking root vegetables, remote controls, chocolate wrappers, fairy lights – or indeed anything else that's irretrievable and inanimate (or, god help us, animate) – up your internal cavities for one day a year. It's only twenty-four hours, guys, and you'll make all their Christmases come at once.

---

* I'm an ambassador for the wonderful Lullaby Trust, who support families bereaved of babies and young children, and fund research into infant death. Any size of donation makes a real difference to their crucial work.

Acknowledgements

To my most fantastic editor, Francesca Main. Without you, terrible nonsense.

To my peerless, fearless and oh-my-god-so-tolerant agents, Cath Summerhayes and Jess Cooper. Without you, chaos.

To my husband, James – the cleverest, most handsome, most annoying, most wonderful person I know. Without you, nothing.

To everyone who bought my last book and those who stuck around for the difficult second album. More of an EP, I guess? To every bookshop, book-seller and library who got it to the readers.

To my family, especially my grandma, who I wish I'd thanked in my last book so she could have seen it. Drifting in and out of lucidity in her final days, she asked how it had sold. When I said it had done well, she replied, 'Maybe the Great British public aren't so stupid after all.' To Naomi and Stewart; Marc, Shazia, Noah and Zareen; Dan, Annie, Lenny and Sidney; Sophie and Rauri.

To Steph von Reiswitz for the inventive, ingenious illustrations. I adore them.

To the amazing help, reminders, and reassurances from Drs Gibson, Heeps, Jones, Wozniak, van Hegan, Rehman, Laycock, Hughes-Roberts, Biswas, Bayliss, Webster and Knight.

To everyone involved in taking *This is Going to Hurt* to stage and screen – especially James Seabright, Annie Cullum, Lee Martin, Hannah Godfrey, Naomi de Pear, Holly Pullinger and Jane Featherstone. To word wizards Justin Myers, Karl Webster and Dan Swimer.

To my publicity supergroup of Dusty Miller and Emma Bravo.

To my uniquely supportive friend Mo Khan, who speaks at international medical conferences and ends every lecture by plugging my books. To Susie Dent for telling me it was OK to keep the word 'tatterdemalion'.

To the dozens of people on the credits pages that follow. I'm proud to join the small band of authors who formally recognize every single person involved in making a book happen. One day this will be standard practice rather than something new and 'quirky'. Also, it really helps with the word count.

EDITORIAL

Publisher Paul Baggaley
Editor and Associate Publisher Francesca Main
Assistant Editor Gillian Fitzgerald-Kelly
Editorial Administrative Assistant Roshani Moorjani

MANAGEMENT

Managing Director Anthony Forbes-Watson
Sales and Brand Director Anna Bond
International Director Jonathan Atkins
Finance Director Lara Borlenghi
Publisher, Macmillan Adult Books Jeremy Trevathan
Digital and Communications Director Sara Lloyd
Publishing Operations Director James Long

FINANCE

Finance Director, Adult Publishing Jo Mower

CONTRACTS

Head of Contracts Clare Miller
Senior Contracts Executive Marta Dziurosz

AUDIO

Audio Publishing Director Rebecca Lloyd
Audio Publishing Executive Laura Marlow

EDITORIAL MANAGEMENT

Associate Publisher Sophie Brewer
Managing Editor Laura Carr
Junior Desk Editor Chloe May
Copy-Editors Charlotte Atyeo, Penny Isaac

Proofreader Fraser Crichton
Editorial Consultant Justin Myers
Medical Advisor Caroline Knight

DESIGN

Art and Design Director James Annal
Design Manager Ami Smithson
Jacket Photograph and Product Designer Kiseung Lee
Author Photograph Idil Sukan
Illustrator Stephanie von Reiswitz
Studio Manager Lloyd Jones
Artworker Alex Fowler

PRODUCTION

Head of Adult Production Simon Rhodes
Senior Production Controller Charlie Tonner
Production Assistant Giacomo Russo
Text Design Manager Lindsay Nash
Typesetter Palimpsest Book Production Ltd

LEGAL

Head of Legal Annie LaPaz

MARKETING & COMMUNICATIONS

Communications Director, Picador Emma Bravo
Publicist Dusty Miller
Head of Marketing, Picador Katie Bowden
Senior Communications and Events Executive Rachel Mellor
Publicist, Ireland Cormac Kinsella

BRAND MANAGEMENT

Senior Brand Manager Charlotte Williams
Senior Brand Executive Jade Tolley
Brand Assistant Molly Robinson

UK SALES

David Adamson

Richard Baker

Andrew Belshaw

Katie Bradburn

Emily Bromfield

Ruth Brooks

Kate Bullows

Tom Clancy

Sarah Clarke

Stuart Dwyer

Bríd Enright

Julia Finnegan

Richard Green

Lucy Hine

Christine Jones

Lucy Jones

Rebecca Kellaway

Clare Lawler

Gillian MacKay

Holly Martin

Rory O'Brien

Alexandra Payne

Guy Raphael

Siobhan Slattery

Toby Watson

Keren Western

INTERNATIONAL SALES

Rachel Graves

Stacey Hamilton

Daniel Jenkins

Louis Patel

Laura Ricchetti

Emily Scorer

Lucie Uwarow

Leanne Williams

RIGHTS

Rights Director Jon Mitchell
Senior Rights Manager Anna Shora
Rights Manager Emma Winter
Rights Assistant Hannah Dualeh

DIGITAL MARKETING

Marketing and Communications Director Lee Dibble
Senior Metadata and Content Manager Eleanor Jones
Metadata Executive Marisa Davies
Audience Manager Andy Joannou
Digital Publishing Executive Alex Ellis

OPERATIONS

Operations Manager Kerry Pretty
Operations Administrator Josh Craig

PRINTERS

Senior Account Director James Longman
Team Leader Karen Goddard